Lung Cancer

Editor

MARK J. KRASNA

SURGICAL ONCOLOGY CLINICS OF NORTH AMERICA

www.surgonc.theclinics.com

Consulting Editor
NICHOLAS J. PETRELLI

July 2016 • Volume 25 • Number 3

ELSEVIER

1600 John F. Kennedy Boulevard • Suite 1800 • Philadelphia, Pennsylvania, 19103-2899

http://www.theclinics.com

SURGICAL ONCOLOGY CLINICS OF NORTH AMERICA Volume 25, Number 3
July 2016 ISSN 1055-3207, ISBN-13: 978-0-323-44857-4

Editor: John Vassallo (j.vassallo@elsevier.com)
Developmental Editor: Meredith Clinton

Surgical Oncology Clinics of North America (ISSN 1055-3207) is published quarterly by Elsevier Inc., 360 Park Avenue South, New York, NY 10010-1710. Months of publication are January, April, July, and October. Business and Editorial Offices: 1600 John F. Kennedy Blvd., Ste. 1800, Philadelphia, PA 19103-2899. Customer Service Office: 3251 Riverport Lane, Maryland Heights, MO 63043. Periodicals postage paid at New York, NY and additional mailing offices. Subscription prices are $290.00 per year (US individuals), $471.00 (US institutions) $100.00 (US student/resident), $330.00 (Canadian individuals), $596.00 (Canadian institutions), $205.00 (Canadian student/resident), $410.00 (foreign individuals), $596.00 (foreign institutions), and $205.00 (foreign student/resident). Foreign air speed delivery is included in all *Clinics* subscription prices. All prices are subject to change without notice. **POSTMASTER**: Send address changes to *Surgical Oncology Clinics of North America,* Elsevier Health Science Division, Subscription Customer Service, 3251 Riverport Lane, Maryland Heights, MO 63043. **Customer Service: 1-800-654-2452 (US and Canada). 314-447-8871 (outside US and Canada). Fax: 314-447-8029. E-mail: journalscustomerservice-usa@elsevier.com (for print support); journalsonline support-usa@elsevier.com (for online support).**

Reprints. For copies of 100 or more, of articles in this publication, please contact the Commercial Reprints Department, Elsevier Inc., 360 Park Avenue South, New York, New York 10010-1710. Tel. 212-633-3874; Fax: 212-633-3820; E-mail: reprints@elsevier.com.

Surgical Oncology Clinics of North America is covered in *MEDLINE/PubMed (Index Medicus)* and *EMBASE/ Excerpta Medica, Current Contents/Clinical Medicine, and ISI/BIOMED.*

Contributors

CONSULTING EDITOR

NICHOLAS J. PETRELLI, MD, FACS
Bank of America Endowed Medical Director, Helen F. Graham Cancer Center and Research Institute, Christiana Care Health System, Newark, Delaware; Professor of Surgery, Thomas Jefferson University, Philadelphia, Pennsylvania

EDITOR

MARK J. KRASNA, MD, FACS
Corporate Medical Director of Oncology, Clinical Professor of Surgery, Rutgers-Robert Wood Johnson Medical School, Meridian Cancer Care, Jersey Shore University Medical Center, Neptune, New Jersey

AUTHORS

GHULAM ABBAS, MD, MHCM, FACS
Director, Minimally Invasive Thoracic Surgery, Meridian Health, Red Bank, New Jersey

NASSER K. ALTORKI, MD
Professor of Cardiothoracic Surgery, New York-Presbyterian Hospital, Weill Cornell Medicine, New York, New York

THOMAS L. BAUER, MD
Director, Thoracic Surgery; Medical Director, Thoracic Oncology Program, Jersey Shore University Medical Center, Meridian Health, Neptune, New Jersey

DAVID B. BERKHEIM, MD
Department of Surgery, Surgery Resident, Christiana Care Health Systems, Newark, Delaware

RAPHAEL BUENO, MD
Professor of Surgery, Division of Thoracic Surgery, Brigham and Women's Hospital, Harvard Medical School, Boston, Massachusetts

ROBERT J. CERFOLIO, MD, MBA
Professor, JH Estes Endowed Chair for Lung Cancer Research, Division of Cardiothoracic Surgery, University of Alabama-Birmingham Medical Center, Chief of Thoracic Surgery, University of Alabama at Birmingham, Birmingham, Alabama

PAUL K. CHUNG, MD
Attending Physician, Hematology and Oncology, Southern Ocean Medical Center, Meridian Cancer Care, Manahawkin, New Jersey

THOMAS A. D'AMICO, MD
Gary Hock Endowed Professor of Surgery, Chief, Section of General Thoracic Surgery, Duke University Medical Center, Durham, North Carolina

ADNAN DANISH, MD
Medical Director, Radiation Oncology, Meridian Health, Red Bank, New Jersey

JATIN K. DESANI, MD
Attending Physician, Hematology and Oncology, Southern Ocean Medical Center, Meridian Cancer Care, Manahawkin, New Jersey

SHADY M. ELDAIF, MD
Section of Thoracic Surgery, Northside Hospital Cancer Institute, Atlanta, Georgia

ZIV GAMLIEL, MD, FACS
Chief, Thoracic Surgery, Angelos Center for Lung Diseases, MedStar Franklin Square Medical Center, MedStar Harbor Hospital, Baltimore, Maryland

MATTHEW A. GAUDET, MD
Department of Cardiothoracic Surgery, Ochsner Medical Center, New Orleans, Louisiana

RICKY J. HAYWOOD-WATSON, MD, PhD
Michael E. DeBakey Department of General Surgery, Baylor College of Medicine, Houston, Texas

JIE HE, MD
Department of Thoracic Surgery, Cancer Institute and Hospital, Chinese Academy of Medical Sciences, Beijing, China

MICHAEL T. JAKLITSCH, MD
Professor of Surgery, Division of Thoracic Surgery, Brigham and Women's Hospital, Harvard Medical School, Boston, Massachusetts

MARK J. KRASNA, MD, FACS
Corporate Medical Director of Oncology, Clinical Professor of Surgery, Rutgers-Robert Wood Johnson Medical School, Meridian Cancer Care, Jersey Shore University Medical Center, Neptune, New Jersey

YOUSHENG MAO, MD
Department of Thoracic Surgery, Cancer Institute and Hospital, Chinese Academy of Medical Sciences, Beijing, China

DOUGLAS A. MILLER, MD
Jersey Shore University Medical Center, Neptune, New Jersey

EVAN C. NAYLOR, MD
Attending Physician, Hematology and Oncology, Southern Ocean Medical Center, Meridian Cancer Care, Manahawkin, New Jersey

BRADLEY PUA, MD
Assistant Professor of Radiology, Director Lung Cancer Screening Program, New York-Presbyterian Hospital, Weill Cornell Medicine, New York, New York

BRENDON M. STILES, MD
Associate Professor of Cardiothoracic Surgery, New York-Presbyterian Hospital, Weill Cornell Medicine, New York, New York

DAVID J. SUGARBAKER, MD
Professor and Chief, Division of General Thoracic Surgery, Michael E. DeBakey
Department of General Surgery, Director, Lung Institute, Olga Keith Wiess Chair in
Surgery, Baylor College of Medicine, Houston, Texas

ORI WALD, MD, PhD
Instructor, Division of General Thoracic Surgery, Michael E. DeBakey Department of
General Surgery, Baylor College of Medicine, Houston, Texas

BENJAMIN WEI, MD
Assistant Professor, Division of Cardiothoracic Surgery, University of Alabama at
Birmingham Medical Center, Birmingham, Alabama

DING YANG, MD
Department of Thoracic Surgery, Cancer Institute and Hospital, Chinese Academy of
Medical Sciences, Beijing, China

MIN ZHENG, MD, PhD
Vice Chair, Department of Pathology, Jersey Shore University Medical Center, Neptune,
New Jersey

YIFAN ZHENG, MD
Clinical Research Fellow, Division of Thoracic Surgery, Brigham and Women's Hospital,
Harvard Medical School, Boston, Massachusetts

Contents

Yousheng Mao, Ding Yang, Jie He, and Mark J. Krasna

> Lung cancer has transformed from a rare disease into a global problem and public health issue. The etiologic factors of lung cancer become more complex along with industrialization, urbanization, and environmental pollution around the world. Currently, the control of lung cancer has attracted worldwide attention. Studies on the epidemiologic characteristics of lung cancer and its relative risk factors have played an important role in the tertiary prevention of lung cancer and in exploring new ways of diagnosis and treatment. This article reviews the current evolution of the epidemiology of lung cancer.

Min Zheng

> Advancement in the understanding of lung tumor biology enables continued refinement of lung cancer classification, reflected in the recently introduced 2015 World Health Organization classification of lung cancer. In small biopsy or cytology specimens, special emphasis is placed on separating adenocarcinomas from the other lung cancers to effectively select tumors for targeted molecular testing. In resection specimens, adenocarcinomas are further classified based on architectural pattern to delineate tissue types of prognostic significance. Neuroendocrine tumors are divided into typical carcinoid, atypical carcinoid, small cell carcinoma, and large cell neuroendocrine carcinoma based on a combination of features, especially tumor cell proliferation rate.

Brendon M. Stiles, Bradley Pua, and Nasser K. Altorki

> Lung cancer is a global health burden and is among the most common and deadliest of all malignancies worldwide. The goal of screening programs is to detect tumors in earlier, curable stages, consequently reducing disease-specific mortality. The issue of screening has great relevance to thoracic surgeons, who should play a leading role in the debate over screening and its consequences. The burden is on thoracic surgeons to work in a multidisciplinary setting to guide and treat these patients safely and responsibly, ensuring low morbidity and mortality of potential diagnostic or therapeutic interventions.

The bronchoscope has gone through much advancement from its origin as a thin metal tube. It has become a highly sophisticated tool for clinicians. Both rigid and the flexible bronchoscopes are invaluable in the diagnosis and treatment of non–small cell lung cancer. Treatment of this disease process hinges on accurate diagnosis and lymph node staging. Technologies, such as endobronchial ultrasound, navigational bronchoscopy, and autofluorescence, have improved efficacy of endobronchial diagnosis and sample collection. If a patient is not a candidate for surgery and has a complication from a centrally located mass, the bronchoscope has been used to deliver palliative therapies.

In the absence of distant metastases, lung cancer treatment is determined by the results of mediastinal lymph node staging. Occult mediastinal lymph node metastases can be missed by radiologic and needle-based staging methods. Aggressive staging of mediastinal lymph nodes improves staging accuracy. Improved accuracy of mediastinal lymph node staging results in more appropriate lung cancer treatment. Improved accuracy of mediastinal lymph node staging can improve stage-specific survival from lung cancer.

Lobectomy is the gold standard treatment in operable patients with surgically resectable non–small cell lung cancer. Thoracoscopic lobectomy has emerged as an option for surgeons facile with the technique. Video-assisted thoracoscopic surgery (VATS) is used for a variety of indications, but its efficacy as a reliable oncologic procedure makes it appealing in the treatment of non–small cell lung cancer. Fewer postoperative complications and decreased postoperative pain associated with VATS procedures can lead to shorter lengths of stay and lower overall costs. Thoracoscopic surgery continues to evolve, and uniportal, robot-assisted, and awake thoracoscopic procedures have all shown promising results.

Robotic-assisted pulmonary lobectomy can be considered for patients able to tolerate conventional lobectomy. Contraindications to resection via thoracotomy apply to patients undergoing robotic lobectomy. Team training, familiarity with equipment, troubleshooting, and preparation are critical for successful robotic lobectomy. Robotic lobectomy is associated with decreased rates of blood loss, blood transfusion, air leak, chest tube duration, length of stay, and mortality compared with thoracotomy. Robotic lobectomy offers many of the same benefits in perioperative morbidity and mortality, and additional advantages in optics, dexterity, and surgeon ergonomics as video-assisted thoracic lobectomy. Long-term oncologic efficacy and cost implications remain areas of study.

Lung cancer is the leading cause of cancer deaths and its incidence continues to increase. Emerging therapies as part of a multimodal approach are making more patients eligible for surgical resection. As more surgeons are treating locally advanced non–small cell lung cancer they find themselves recommending pneumonectomy as the surgical component of the multidisciplinary plan. Performing a pneumonectomy is technically demanding and is associated with many potential perioperative comorbidities. With the proper preparation, experience, and attention to perioperative care, pneumonectomy can be carried out safely with excellent outcomes and a good quality of life.

The treatment paradigm for early stage lung cancer and oligometastatic disease to the lung is rapidly changing. Ablative therapies, especially stereotactic body radiation therapy, are challenging the surgical gold standard and have the potential to be the standard for operable patients with early stage lung cancer who are high risk due to co- morbidities. The most commonly used ablative modalities include stereotactic body radiation therapy, microwave ablation, and radiofrequency ablation.

Locally advanced (stage IIIA) non–small cell lung cancer (NSCLC) is confined to the chest, but requires more than surgery to maximize cure. Therapy given preoperatively is termed *neoadjuvant*, whereas postoperative therapy is termed *adjuvant*. Trimodality therapy (chemotherapy, radiation, and surgery) has become the standard treatment regimen for resectable, locally advanced NSCLC. During the past 2 decades, several prospective, randomized, and nonrandomized studies have explored various regimens for preoperative treatment of NSCLC. The evaluation of potential candidates with NSCLC for neoadjuvant therapy as well as the currently available therapeutic regimens are reviewed.

Patients with stage I and stage II non–small cell lung cancer undergoing complete resection have a 40% to 70% 5-year overall survival despite optimal local therapy. Chemotherapy administered after complete resection has been shown to improve overall survival at 5 years by approximately 5%. This improvement in survival may be confined to patients with stage IB disease 4 cm or greater, and to those with hilar or mediastinal lymph node involvement. The optimal chemotherapy regimen appears to be cisplatin-based doublet or triplet chemotherapy for 3 to 4 cycles. The addition of biologic agents has failed to improve outcomes.

Targeted therapy and immunotherapy have changed the treatment paradigm of non–small cell lung cancer (NSCLC). Distinct molecular subtypes of NSCLC have been described over the past 20 years, enabling the emergence of treatments specific to that subtype. Agents targeting the driver mutations in NSCLC have revolutionized the approach to patients with metastatic disease, because oncologists now select a treatment based on the profile of that particular tumor. More recently, an understanding of immune checkpoints has led to the development of checkpoint inhibitors that enable the host immune system to better recognize tumor cells as foreign and to destroy them.

Advances in surgical, radiation, and interventional radiology therapies carry a reduction in morbidity associated with therapy. Aggressive management of patients with oligometastatic non–small cell lung cancer offers the potential for improved disease-free survival and quality of life compared with traditional systemic therapy alone.

SURGICAL ONCOLOGY
CLINICS OF NORTH AMERICA

Foreword

Lung Cancer

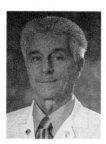

Nicholas J. Petrelli, MD, FACS
Consulting Editor

This issue of the *Surgical Oncology Clinics of North America* is devoted to lung cancer. The guest editor is Mark J Krasna, MD. Dr Krasna is the Medical Director of Meridian Cancer Care. Dr Krasna is a board-certified thoracic surgeon and throughout his career has been an advocate of clinical trials. Prior to his appointment at Meridian, he was a leader in the evolving National Cancer Institute Community Cancer Centers Project, and was a major contributor to the multidisciplinary approach to cancer care.

The American Cancer Society estimates reveal that there will be 158,800 deaths from lung cancer in 2016. These deaths exceed the total deaths from breast cancer (40,890), colorectal cancer (49,190), and prostate cancer (26,120). This issue of the *Surgical Oncology Clinics of North America* covers the gamut of the diagnosis and treatment of lung cancer. There is an excellent article by Drs Y. Zheng, M.T. Jaklitsch, and R. Bueno on neoadjuvant therapy in non–small cell lung cancer, which includes a description of a complete evaluation for patients diagnosed with lung cancer. Drs B. Wei, S.M. Eldaif, and R. Cerfolio have contributed an article entitled, "Robotic Lung Resection for Non–Small Cell Lung Cancer." This discussion includes a comparison of robotic lobectomy versus video-assisted thoracic surgery. A third article by Drs E.C. Naylor, J.K. Desani, and P.K. Chung from Meridian Health discusses targeted therapy and immunotherapy for lung cancer, which has made a major impact in recent years in the treatment of patients with lung cancer. Drs B.M. Stiles, B. Pua, and N.K. Altorki discuss screening for lung cancer, which, with the use of low-dose CT scans, has demonstrated a decrease in lung cancer mortality. Last, Drs T. Bauer and D. Berkheim have a detailed article on diagnostic and therapeutic bronchoscopy for non–small cell lung cancer. This article includes a description of endobronchial ultrasound and electromagnetic navigational bronchoscopy.

The last time the *Surgical Oncology Clinics of North America* devoted an issue to lung cancer was in 2011. Under the guidance of Dr Krasna, the 2016 issue

Surg Oncol Clin N Am 25 (2016) xiii–xiv
http://dx.doi.org/10.1016/j.soc.2016.03.001
1055-3207/16/$ – see front matter © 2016 Published by Elsevier Inc.

surgonc.theclinics.com

demonstrates how far the diagnosis and treatment of lung cancer have come in just five years. I'd like to thank Dr Krasna and his colleagues for updating our readers on this very important and timely subject.

Nicholas J. Petrelli, MD, FACS
Helen F. Graham Cancer Center and
Research Institute
Christiana Care Health System
4701 Ogletown-Stanton Road, Suite 1233
Newark, DE 19713, USA

E-mail address:
npetrelli@christianacare.org

Preface

Lung Cancer

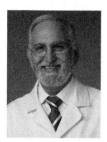

Mark J. Krasna, MD
Editor

Welcome to the *Surgical Oncology Clinics of North America*. This issue has been dedicated to an update on Lung Cancer, and again, I thank the series editor, Dr Nicholas Petrelli, for being such a close friend and mentor over the last 20 years. Much has changed in lung cancer since 2011, and I am delighted to be joined by a panel of national and international experts on this disease, which still accounts for the majority of the cancer death burden in the United States, and in many developed countries abroad. Although legislation and regulations have had some effect on smoking, overall, the marketing of cigarettes and other tobacco products has continued to grow and shift with an international approach. Improved product labeling and new warnings, as is done in India, where a warning sign flashes on the screen before a scene with cigar smoking, are exceptional ideas of progress but not yet the rule. We therefore are still reaping the terrible yield of tobacco-related cancer and cancer deaths even now, several generations after it was first identified as a carcinogen.

The Epidemiology of Lung Cancer is presented this time by Dr Yousheng Mao. He is a distinguished professor and chairman of thoracic malignancies at the renowned Chinese Academy of Science Cancer Center. His review is timely in exposing the current shift in epidemiology of lung cancer from smokers to include nonsmokers, from men to women, and from the developed countries to developing countries. One of the greatest changes since the last issue in 2011 is the recognition of the value of computed tomography (CT) screening for lung cancer. Dr Nasser Altorki and colleagues have been at the forefront of the randomized trials to determine the benefit of CT screening. Their thoughtful review of the current data explains the new decisions regarding coverage for this test among certain groups of patients identified as "high risk." Pathology of lung cancer has undergone huge changes in definitions (by the WHO) as well as in modifications on reporting based on revisions to the new staging system (endorsed by the International Association for the Study of Lung Cancer). Dr Min Zheng, who has worked with me hand in hand in

Surg Oncol Clin N Am 25 (2016) xv–xvii
http://dx.doi.org/10.1016/j.soc.2016.03.002
1055-3207/16/$ – see front matter © 2016 Published by Elsevier Inc.

launching the thoracic oncology program at Meridian Health, has done a remarkable job of presenting the field in a clear and concise way.

The staging of lung cancer is crucial, and after ruling out distant metastases, mediastinal staging for lung cancer is of utmost importance in determining whether surgery alone or a combined modality approach should be used. This is presented by my former partner, Dr Ziv Gamliel, currently chief of Thoracic Surgery at MedStar Health. Bronchoscopy as both a diagnostic and a therapeutic tool has become indispensable for non–small cell lung cancer (NSCLC). Dr Thomas Bauer, the new Medical Director for Thoracic Oncology at Meridian, has been a champion of these newer techniques, including endobronchial ultrasound and electromagnetic navigation bronchoscopy, and describes their place in the armamentarium for the thoracic surgeons.

The standard surgical approach to resectable lesions remains lobectomy. Although the most common approach across the nation remains open thoracotomy, video-assisted thoroscopic surgery lobectomy for NSCLC has clearly been shown to be equal as an oncologic procedure and beneficial from the perspective of patient discomfort and loss of work. I'm delighted that Dr Thomas D'Amico, who has trained many of the surgeons in the world, and who adopted this procedure early on, has agreed to present his clear, thoughtful, step-by-step technical approach to this procedure, whose time has clearly come. Robotic lung resection for NSCLC is now the next "big" thing in thoracic surgery. Dr Robert Cerfolio has done more to champion this technique with a technical and team approach and shares his system herein.

Pneumonectomy for NSCLC is being used less and less as we all take a lung-sparing approach to patients with a view to cure and long-term survival; however, technical and anatomic situations occur regularly and require the thoracic surgeon to be proficient. Dr David Sugarbaker not only has described this in patients with mesothelioma, but also has had some of the best data in NSCLC as well, including operating on patients after neoadjuvant therapy with chemo and/or radiation.

Whereas in the past, surgery was seen as curative for only a small number of patients with lung cancer, the use of neoadjuvant therapy for lung cancer has allowed the surgeon to include the multimodality team prospectively and utilize chemotherapy and/or radiation therapy prior to resection to achieve mediastinal clearance and cure. Dr Raphael Bueno has written extensively on this field and shares the excellent results from the Brigham Group.

Alternative treatments for patients with local regional lung cancer have evolved. Data now exist on the use of stereotactic body radiation therapy as well as other ablative therapies for NSCLC. These are presented by Dr Adnan Danish, from radiation oncology, and Dr Ghulam Abbas, from thoracic surgery, who show how approaching these lesions as a team allows us to determine the right intervention for the right patient.

Dr Douglas Miller, who has led our effort to bring academics and new trials in radiation oncology to Meridian Health, has joined me in describing the current status of treatment of patients with oligometastatic disease for NSCLC.

Adjuvant therapy for local regional NSCLC has become established as part of the routine approach to cure this disease. Making lung cancer care a true team sport, by use of either adjuvant or neoadjuvant therapy in stage I, II, and III NSCLC, has become a new norm. The choice of agents supported by guidelines has now shifted to molecular/targeted therapy for lung cancer based on histology and specific expression of molecular targets. Dr Naylor and colleagues describe how this has given rise to a new generation of treatments that are linked to specific tests to be done prior to beginning therapy.

I hope you enjoy this issue and find the information exciting and up-to-date.

Mark J. Krasna, MD
Rutgers-Robert Wood Johnson Medical School
Jersey Shore University Medical Center
Ackerman South-Room 553
1945 Route 33
Neptune, NJ 07753, USA

E-mail address:
mkrasna@meridianhealth.com

Epidemiology of Lung Cancer

Yousheng Mao, MD[a], Ding Yang, MD[a], Jie He, MD[a],*, Mark J. Krasna, MD[b],*

KEYWORDS

• Lung cancer • Epidemiology • Etiology

KEY POINTS

• Lung cancer is the most frequent malignant tumor with the highest mortality around the world.
• Recent epidemic studies found that tobacco use, radon exposure, indoor and outdoor air pollution, relative harmful occupational exposure, hereditary susceptibility, radiation exposure, and unbalanced diet are responsible for the increase in lung cancer incidence.
• These findings can assist us in preventing lung cancer from the etiologic level. Effective and practical public health policy such as tobacco use restriction law, air pollution control, and antismoking education of teenagers should be established to decrease the lung cancer incidence.

EPIDEMIOLOGIC CHARACTERISTICS
Incidence and Mortality

Globally, lung cancer is the most common cancer and the leading cause of cancer death in men and is the third most common cancer (after breast and colorectal cancers) and the second leading cause of cancer death (after breast cancer) in women. About 1.8 million new cases of lung cancer were diagnosed in 2012, which accounted for 12.9% of the world's total cancer incidence. The worldwide lung cancer mortality rate amounted to 1.59 million deaths in 2012,[1] accounting for 19.4% of the total cancer deaths.

Smoking is a known major risk factor for lung cancer, so lung cancer epidemiologic trends, and its variations, reflect the past trends of cigarette smoking to a great extent. In the United States, most states drew up legislation for smoking restrictions in public areas about 20 years ago and have continually promoted the awareness of smoking hazards to their residents.[2] Many states have passed the peak of the tobacco-related epidemic; therefore, both the incidence and mortality rates of lung cancer in these areas are decreasing.[3]

The authors have nothing to disclose.
[a] Department of Thoracic Surgery, Cancer Institute and Hospital, Chinese Academy of Medical Sciences, Beijing 100021, China; [b] Meridian Cancer Care, Jersey Shore University Medical Center, Ackerman South-Room 553, 1945 Route 33, Neptune City, NJ 07753, USA
* Corresponding authors.
E-mail addresses: prof.hejie@263.net; MKrasna@meridianhealth.com

Over the last several decades, the incidence of adenocarcinoma of the lung has increased more rapidly than that of squamous cell carcinoma in men and especially in women.[4] Adenocarcinoma has become the most common histologic cancer type diagnosed around the world since 2004, according to statistics from the World Health Organization.[5] This trend probably is associated with the change of historic pattern of tobacco use or the smoke of modern filtered cigarettes.[4] Sex differences in lung cancer mortality patterns also reflect historical differences between men and women in the increase and reduction of cigarette smoking over the last 50 years.

In developing countries such as China, not only the incidence but also the mortality rate of lung cancer has been increasing rapidly; incidence was ranked first in men and second in women; however, the death rate ranked first in both men and women from the annual report of the China national cancer registration.[6] The adenocarcinoma subtype has become the major pathologic type not only in the nonsmoking population but also in the smoking population. The smoking pattern, therefore, may be changing but may only be a partial cause of the pathologic evolution of lung cancer. Lung cancer incidence may be related to air pollution caused by rapid and immature industrialization and continual increased use of automobiles in cities.

The global geographic distribution of lung cancer shows marked regional variation. In men, the highest incidence rates are observed in Central and Eastern Europe (53.5 per 100,000) and Eastern Asia (50.4 per 100,000). Notably low incidence rates are observed in Middle and Western Africa (2.0 and 1.7 per 100,000, respectively). In women, the incidence rates are generally lower, and the geographic pattern is a little different, mainly reflecting different historical exposure to tobacco smoking. Thus, the highest estimated rates are in Northern America (33.8) and Northern Europe (23.7) with a relatively high rate in Eastern Asia (19.2) and the lowest rates again in Western and Middle Africa (1.1 and 0.8, respectively). For lung cancer mortality, because of its high fatality (the overall ratio of mortality to incidence is 0.87) and the relative lack of variability in survival in different world regions, the geographic patterns in mortality closely follow those in incidence.

Incidence and mortality rates of lung cancer also differ by ethnicity. In 2012, black Americans had the highest incidence rates of 62 per 100,000 and the highest mortality rates of 48.4 per 100,000, whereas Hispanics had the lowest rate of 28 per 100,000 in incidence and the lowest rate of 19.4 per 100,000 in mortality.[7]

Survival

The incidence and mortality rates of lung cancer tend to mirror one another because most patients with lung cancer eventually die of it.[8] Despite the new diagnostic and genetic technologies that are now available and the many advances in surgical technique and biologic treatment, such as targeted treatment and immunotherapy, the overall 5-year survival rate (2005–2011) of lung cancer in the United States is still dismal (17.4%).[7] The global situation is also worse than before.[8] Most lung cancer is discovered at an advanced stage, and the fact that only 15% of lung cancers are discovered in early stages may be responsible for the dismal prognosis.[9] Therefore, early diagnosis by screening high-risk populations using low-dose computed tomography scan and effective biomarkers may improve the survival of lung cancer patients.[10–12]

RISK FACTORS
Tobacco

The prevalence of lung cancer has been confirmed as a consequence of the widespread addiction to cigarettes throughout the world.[1] Many developed countries have now passed the peak of the tobacco-related epidemic, and their lung cancer incidence and mortality rates are decreasing.[7]

As a single etiologic agent, tobacco is by far the most important risk factor in the development of lung cancer. It is estimated that around the world, 80% of lung cancer cases in men and 50% in women each year are caused by smoking.[3] The abundance of evidence of dose-response relationship and biological plausibility overwhelmingly supports the existence of a causal relationship between smoking and lung cancer.[13] The same relationship exists between passive smoking (so-called second-hand smoke) and lung cancer.[14,15]

The risk for lung cancer among cigarette smokers increases along with long duration of smoking; some studies showed stronger effect of smoking duration than smoking amount per day.[16] Young smokers have a greater likelihood of becoming heavier smokers and maintain their smoking habit, and the risk of suffering lung cancer by long and heavy smoking remarkably increases. Therefore, antismoking campaigns aimed at teenagers are obviously necessary and effective in reducing lung cancer risk. Meanwhile, cigarette smokers can decrease their risk of lung cancer development by quitting smoking at any age.[17]

Recent research finds that smoking filtered cigarettes can decrease tar absorption but can increase intake of nitrosamines. It may be one of the important factors resulting in the pathologic change from squamous cell carcinoma into adenocarcinoma.[4]

Air Pollution

Outdoor or indoor air pollution is a significant environmental risk factor for lung cancer; long-term exposure to polluted air caused by factories and automobiles, cooking fumes, or formaldehyde from indoor decoration definitely increases the risk of lung cancer.[18] Early ecologic studies found that more than 50% of lung cancer occurred in urban areas, which is most probably more from polluted air from industrial sources and vehicle exhaust than in rural areas. A series of case-control and cohort studies found a notable association between lung cancer and air pollution with adequate adjustment for tobacco use and other potential risk factors.[19–26]

Outdoor air pollution mostly comes from vehicle exhaust, heating systems, and industrial burning waste. Carcinogens that are generated by combustion of fossil fuels include polycyclic aromatic hydrocarbons and metals such as arsenic, nickel, and chromium.[27] A recent study also indicates that mono-nitrogen oxides nitric oxide and nitrogen dioxide are the main carcinogenic agents from vehicle exhaust.[18] Study results from Liaw and colleagues[28] showed that there was a dose-response relationship between gaseous nitric oxide concentrations and lung adenocarcinoma.[28] A study by Yu and colleagues[29] found the mutation spectrum of air pollution–related lung cancers and provided evidence of an air pollution exposure–genomic mutation relationship on a large scale.

Indoor air pollution includes cooking fumes, formaldehyde and benzene from decorative and building materials, and environmental tobacco smoke. According to the Ministry of Health of China, women and children are more likely to be the victims of indoor air pollution, as they spend most of their time indoors.[30] Epidemiologic studies found that lung cancer incidence increases with the number of meals cooked per day; exposure to fumes from cooking oils is an important risk factor for lung cancer in rural China.[31,32] From the research carried out in Xuanwei County, China over several decades, household coal use is the major source of household air pollution; the studies also identified that household coal fuel use contributed to the high mortality rate of lung cancer in this region.[33]

Radon

Radon is an inert gas that is produced naturally from radium in the decay series of uranium.[13] Indoor radon concentrations usually come from the soil and building materials. Radon is likely the second most common cause of lung cancer after smoking; about 20,000 lung cancer deaths each year in the United States are radon related.[34] Three cohort studies conducted in the Europe, North America, and China, found that chronic exposure to radon contributes to the occurrence of lung cancer. The relative risk of lung cancer in the observed radon concentration greater than per 100 Bq/m^3 was 8% (95 confidence interval [CI], 3%–6%), 11% (95 CI, 0%–28%), and 13% (95 CI, 1%–36%), respectively.[35–37]

Occupational Exposure

The International Agency for Research on Cancer has identified 12 occupational exposure factors as being carcinogenic to the human lung (aluminum production, arsenic, asbestos, bis-chloromethyl ether, beryllium, cadmium, hexavalent chromium, coke and coal gasification fumes, crystalline silica, nickel, radon, and soot).[38–40] Asbestos is a well-established occupational carcinogen and refers to several forms of fibrous, naturally occurring silicate minerals; exposure to asbestos at high levels can cause lung cancer and mesothelioma.[9] From cohort studies on cancer mortality among workers exposed to asbestos in China, a significantly elevated meta–standard mortality ratio for lung cancer is 4.54, with 95% CI of 2.49 to 8.24.[41] Concurrent smoking and asbestos exposure are synergistic and result in increased cancer incidence.

Hereditary Susceptibility

Most studies indicate that more than 80% of lung cancer occurrence is associated with the habit of smoking, but less than 20% of smokers will have lung cancer, which suggests that lung cancer occurrence probably possesses genetic susceptibility.[3] Forty years ago, Tokuhata and Lilienfeld[42] provided the first epidemiologic evidence of familial aggregation of lung cancer. Studies find that the lung cancer risk of the probands' first-degree relatives was 1.88 times higher than that of the controls' families.[43] Several novel lung cancer susceptibility genes have been identified by recent large-scale genomewide association studies, including those on chromosomes 5p15.33, 6p21,15q24 to 25.1,6q23 to 25, and 13q31.3.[44] The risk of disease can be conceptualized as reflecting the joint consequences of the interrelationship between exposure to etiologic agents and the individual susceptibility to these agents.[45] For lung cancer, some relevance of gene environment have been identified. For example, the 15q25 region contains 3 nicotine acetylcholine receptor subunit genes, and nicotine addiction is indirectly associated with lung cancer risk by increase of tobacco carcinogen intake. Meanwhile, this gene is also identified as a risk factor for several smoking-related diseases, such as chronic obstructive pulmonary disease. Furthermore, there are still several other molecular pathways for the development of lung adenocarcinomas, such as the 5p15.33, but their mechanism are still unclear.[44]

Radiation

Two types of radiation are relevant to lung cancer: low linear energy transfer radiation (eg, x-rays, gamma rays) and high linear energy transfer radiation (eg, neutrons, radon). Epidemiologic studies find that exposure to high doses of radiation is associated with lung cancer. However, whether low-dose radiation is relevant to lung cancer is still unclear.[46]

Diet

After decades of research on diet and lung cancer, many specific micronutrients thought to have anticarcinogenic activity, such as retinol and beta-carotene, have been found. Most of the micronutrients are common in fruits and vegetables.[47,48] Intake of more fresh fruits and vegetables may decrease the risk of lung cancer.

Others

There are still other risk factors for lung cancer, such as human immunodeficiency virus infection and estrogen levels; the question of whether these factors are real risk factors for lung cancer has been controversial, and further studies are needed to evaluate this conclusively.

SUMMARY

Lung cancer is the most frequent malignant tumor with high mortality around the world. Recent epidemic studies find that tobacco use, radon exposure, indoor and outdoor air pollution, relative harmful occupational exposure, hereditary susceptibility, radiation exposure, and unbalanced diet are responsible for the increasing lung cancer incidence. These findings can assist us in preventing lung cancer from the etiologic level. Effective and practical public health policy such as tobacco use restriction law, air pollution control, and antismoking education of teenagers should be established to decrease the lung cancer incidence.

REFERENCES

1. Ferlay J, Soerjomataram I, Ervik M, et al. GLOBOCAN 2012 v1.0, Cancer incidence and mortality Worldwide: IARC CancerBase No. 11 [Internet]. Lyon (France): International Agency for Research on Cancer; 2013. Available at: http://globocan.iarc.fr.
2. Fishman JA, Allison H, Knowles SB, et al. State laws on tobacco control–United States, 1998. MMWR CDC Surveill Summ 1999;48(3):21–40.
3. Jemal A, Bray F, Center MM, et al. Global cancer statistic. CA Cancer J Clin 2011; 61(2):69–90.
4. Stellman SD, Muscat JE, Thompson S, et al. Risk of squamous cell carcinoma and adenocarcinoma of the lung in relation to lifetime filter cigarette smoking. Cancer 1997;80(3):382–8.
5. Beasley MB, Brambilla E, Travis WD. The 2004 World Health Organization classification of lung tumors. Semin Roentgenol 2005;40(2):90–7.
6. He J, Chen WQ. Chinese cancer registry annual report 2012. Beijing (China): Military Medical Science Press; 2012.
7. Howlader N, Noone AM, Krapcho M, et al, editors. SEER Cancer statistics review, 1975-2012. Bethesda (MD): National Cancer Institute; 2015. Available at: http://seer.cancer.gov/csr/1975_2012/.
8. Dela Cruz CS, Tanoue LT, Matthay RA, et al. Lung cancer: epidemiology, etiology, and prevention. Clin Chest Med 2011;32(4):605–44.
9. Ridge CA, McErlean AM, Ginsberg MS. Epidemiology of lung cancer. Semin Intervent Radiol 2013;30:93–8.
10. Eberth JM. Lung cancer screening with low-dose CT in the United States. J Am Coll Radiol 2015;12(12 Pt B):1395–402.

11. Guldbrandt LM, Fenger GM, Rasmussen TR, et al. The effect of direct access to CT scan in early lung cancer detection: an unblinded, cluster-randomised trial. BMC Cancer 2015;15(1):934.

12. Kumar V, Becker K, Zheng HX, et al. The performance of NLST screening criteria in Asian lung cancer patients. BMC Cancer 2015;15(1):916.

13. Alberg AJ, Ford JG, Samet JM. Epidemiology of lung cancer: ACCP evidence - based clinical practice guidelines (2nd edition). Chest 2007;132(3 Suppl): 29S–55S.

14. The health consequences of involuntary smoking: a report of the Surgeon General. Washington, DC: US Government Printing Office, US Department of Health and Human Services; 1986. p. 87–8398.

15. Respiratory health effects of passive smoking: lung cancer and other disorders. Washington, DC: US Government Printing Office, US Environmental Protection Agency; 1992. publication EPA/600/600F.

16. Peto R. Influence of dose and duration of smoking on lung cancer rates. In: Zaridze D, Peto R, editors. Tobacco: a major international health hazard; proceedings of an international meeting, June 4–6, 1985, Moscow, vol. 74. Lyon (France): World Health Organization, International Agency for Research on Cancer, IARC Science Publication; 1986. p. 23–33.

17. Centers for Disease Control (CDC). Smoking and health: a national status report. MMWR Morb Mortal Wkly Rep 1986;35(46):709–11.

18. Raaschou - Nielsen O, Bak H, Sorensen M, et al. Air pollution from traffic and risk for lung cancer in three Danish cohorts. Cancer Epidemiol Biomarkers Prev 2010; 19(5):1284.

19. Dockery DW, Pope CA III, Xu X, et al. An association between air pollution and mortality in six U.S. Cities. N Engl J Med 1993;329(24):1753–9.

20. Beeson WL, Abbey DE, Knutsen SF, et al. Adventist Health Study on Smog. Long-term concentrations of ambient air pollutants and incident lung cancer in California adults: results from the AHSMOG study. Environ Health Perspect 1998; 106(12):813–23.

21. Pope CA III, Burnett RT, Thun MJ, et al. Lung cancer, cardiopulmonary mortality, and long-term exposure to fine particulate air pollution. JAMA 2002;287(9): 1132–41.

22. Nyberg F, Gustavsson P, Jarup L, et al. Urban air pollution and lung cancer in Stockholm. Epidemiology 2000;11(5):487–95.

23. Nafstad P, Haheim LL, Oftedal B, et al. Lung cancer and air pollution: a 27 year follow up of 16 209 Norwegian men. Thorax 2003;58(12):1071–6.

24. Vineis P, Hoek G, Krzyzanowski M, et al. Air pollution and risk of lung cancer in a prospective study in Europe. Int J Cancer 2006;119(1):169–74.

25. Beelen R, Hoek G, van den Brandt PA, et al. Long-term exposure to traffic-related air pollution and lung cancer risk. Epidemiology 2008;19(5):702–10.

26. Yorifuji T, Kashima S, Tsuda T, et al. Long-term exposure to trafficrelated air pollution and mortality in Shizuoka, Japan. Occup Environ Med 2010;67(2):111–7.

27. Alberg AJ, Yung R, Strickland PT, et al. Respiratory cancer and exposure to arsenic, chromium, nickel and polycyclic aromatic hydrocarbons. Clin Occup Environ Med 2002;2(4):779–801.

28. Liaw YP, Ting TF, Ho CC, et al. Cell type specificity of lung cancer associated with nitric oxide. Sci Total Environ 2010;208(41):4931–4.

29. Yu XJ, Yang MJ, Zhou B, et al. Characterization of somatic mutations in air pollution-related lung cancer. EBioMedicine 2015;2(6):583–90.

30. Zhang YP, Mo JH, Weschler CJ. Reducing health risks from indoor exposures in rapidly developing urban China. Environ Health Perspect 2013;121(7):751–5.
31. Wu-Williams AH, Da XD, Blot W, et al. Lung cancer among women in north-east China. Br J Cancer 1990;62(6):982–7.
32. Liu Q, Sasco AJ, Riboli E, et al. Indoor air pollution and lung cancer in Guangzhou, People's Republic of China. Am J Epidemiol 1993;137(2):145–54.
33. Lan Q, Chapman RS, Schreinemachers DM, et al. Household stove improvement and risk of lung cancer in Xuanwei, China. J Natl Cancer Inst 2002;94(11): 826–35.
34. Pawel DJ, Puskin JS. The U.S. Environmental Protection Agency's assessment of risks from indoor radon. Health Phys 2004;87(1):68–74.
35. Darby S, Hill D, Deo H, et al. Residential radon and lung cancer–detailed results of a collaborative analysis of individual data on 7148 persons with lung cancer and 14,208 persons without lung cancer from 13 epidemiologic studies in Europe. Scand J Work Environ Health 2006;32(Suppl 1):1–83.
36. Krewski D, Lubin JH, Zielinski JM, et al. A combined analysis of North American case-control studies of residential radon and lung cancer. J Toxicol Environ Health A 2006;69(7):533–97.
37. Lubin JH, Zuo Yuan W, Boice JD, et al. Risk of lung cancer and residential radon in China: pooled results of two studies. Int J Cancer 2004;109(1):132–7.
38. International Agency for Research on Cancer. Overall evaluations of carcinogenicity: an updating of IARC monographs volumes 1 to 42. IARC Monogr Eval Carcinog Risks Hum Suppl 1987;7:1–440.
39. IARC Working Group on the Evaluation of Carcinogenic Risks to Humans:Silica, Some Silicates, Coal Dust and Para-Aramid Fibrils. Lyon, 15-22 October 1996. IARC Monogr Eval Carcinog Risks Hum 1997;68:1–475.
40. Steenland K, Loomis D, Shy C, et al. Review of occupational lung carcinogens. Am J Ind Med 1996;29(5):474–90.
41. Sun TD, Chen JE, Zhang XJ, et al. Cohort studies on cancer mortality among workers exposed to asbestos in China: a Meta-analysis. Chin Occup Med 2006;33(4):257–9.
42. Tokuhata GK, Lilienfeld AM. Familial aggregation of lung cancer among hospital patients. Public Health Rep 1963;78(4):277–84.
43. Gu J, Hua F, Zhong D, et al. Systematic review of the relationship between family history of lung cancer and lung cancer risk. Zhongguo Fei Ai Za Zhi 2010;13(3): 224–9 [in Chinese].
44. Yokota J, Shiraishi K, Kohno T. Genetic basis for susceptibility to lung cancer: recent progress and future directions. Adv Cancer Res 2010;109:51–72.
45. White C, Bailar JC III. Retrospective and prospective methods of studying association in medicine. Am J Public Health 1956;46(1):35–44.
46. Hendee WR. Estimation of radiation risks: BEIR V and its significance for medicine. JAMA 1992;268(5):620–4.
47. Peto R, Doll R, Buckley JD, et al. Can dietary beta-carotene materially reduce human cancer rates? Nature 1981;290(5803):201–8.
48. Alberg AJ, Samet JM. Epidemiology of lung cancer. In: Sadler MJ, Caballero B, Strain JJ, editors. Encyclopedia of human nutrition. London: Academic Press; 2005. p. 272–84.

Classification and Pathology of Lung Cancer

Min Zheng, MD, PhD

KEYWORDS

- Lung cancer • Classification • Pathology • Immunohistochemistry
- Molecular testing

KEY POINTS

- Lung cancer classification strives to correlate tumor cell morphology with tumor biological characteristics, thus facilitating therapeutic decision-making and effective prognostic outcome prediction in the era of personalized medicine.
- In small biopsy specimens or cytology specimens, major types of lung cancers are established by morphologic evaluation, that is, adenocarcinoma and squamous cell carcinoma.
- When poorly differentiated carcinomas are encountered, judicious application of immunohistochemical stains facilitates such distinction in most cases.
- In resection specimens, lung adenocarcinomas are further divided into low-grade (lepidic adenocarcinoma), intermediate-grade (acinar and papillary adenocarcinomas), and high-grade (solid and micropapillary adenocarcinomas) types of prognostic significance.
- Analysis of neuroendocrine tumors is initiated by the recognition of neuroendocrine morphology, verified by neuroendocrine marker expression when necessary.

INTRODUCTION

Significant progress has been made in the understanding of lung cancer biology, due in large part to advancement in the understanding of tumor biology and pathogenesis. Acquisition of key somatic mutations acts as a sentinel event in lung carcinogenesis, essential for tumor cell growth and division.[1] Molecular detection of driver mutations in specific histologic types of lung cancer can predict favorable response to targeted therapy. The essence of personalized medicine is to tailor individual lung cancer treatment based on accurate histologic classification and biomarker information. Therefore, characterization of histologic type of lung cancer plays an increasingly pivotal role in the multidisciplinary approach in the diagnosis and management of lung cancer. Recognizing the biological diversity of lung cancer, a comprehensive and accurate tumor classification has been developed, which is important for treatment and prognosis. Pathology of lung cancer has expanded to cover both tissue diagnosis

The author has nothing to disclose.
Department of Pathology, Jersey Shore University Medical Center, 1945 Route 33, Neptune, NJ 07753, USA
E-mail address: mzheng@meridianhealth.com

and selection of specific subtypes of lung cancers for further molecular testing. Confirmatory histologic diagnosis directs surgical resection of early-stage disease, whereas pathologic classification and molecular testing enable selection of tumor type–tailored adjuvant therapy and genotype-based treatment regimen to improve the survivals of advanced-stage patients.

Lung cancers are traditionally divided into non–small cell carcinoma (NSCC) and small cell carcinoma (small cell lung carcinoma, SCLC), with the former accounting for 80% of the cases and the latter accounting for the remaining 20%. SCLCs behave aggressively and are treated nonsurgically in most cases, whereas NSCCs are managed by a combination of surgery and adjuvant therapy. Recognition of the diversity of NSCC has led to its subclassification, culminating in the 2004 and 2015 World Health Organization (WHO) classifications.[2,3] Major types of NSCC include adenocarcinoma, squamous cell carcinoma (SSC), and large cell carcinoma (LCC). Thus, subtype of NSCC is specified, whereas the designation "NSCC" is only preserved in certain small biopsies and cytology specimens. SCLC is grouped with other tumors exhibiting neuroendocrine differentiation. Since the publication of the last volume, significant update in lung cancer classification has occurred for lung adenocarcinomas based on better understanding of tumor biology. This update is manifested by streamlined classification for small biopsies and cytology specimens, with special emphasis on separating adenocarcinomas from the rest of the lung cancers in order to effectively screen cases responsive to current mutation-driven therapeutic paradigms. More detailed histologic subtyping is used in resection specimens to delineate tissue types of prognostic significance. This article discusses current pathologic classification of lung cancer, with an emphasis on updating readers to the new WHO lung adenocarcinoma classification (**Box 1**).[3] This article thus serves as a springboard for effective surgical and medical treatment modalities discussed in other articles in this series.

ADENOCARCINOMA

Adenocarcinoma is the most common type of lung cancer, accounting for more than 40% of lung cancers, 60% of the NSCC, and more than 70% of surgically resected cases.[3,4] The incidence of adenocarcinoma has risen steadily over the past few decades. Lung adenocarcinoma commonly forms a peripherally located mass with central fibrosis and pleural puckering. It can also have a variety of other gross appearances, including centrally located mass, diffuse lobar consolidation, bilateral multinodular distribution, and pleural thickening. By definition, lung adenocarcinoma is a malignant epithelial neoplasm with glandular differentiation or mucin production. When such morphologic features are recognized, the tumor can be designated as adenocarcinoma, even in small biopsy specimens. Lung adenocarcinoma cells usually express pneumocytic markers. Thyroid transcription factor (TTF-1) and NapsinA are expressed in more than 85% of the lung adenocarcinoma cases and thus can serve as markers of adenocarcinoma or adenocarcinoma differentiation in poorly differentiated tumor and in limited biopsy sampling material (**Fig. 1**).[5–7] Tumor classification based on ancillary tests such as immunohistochemistry (IHC) is designated as "NSCC, favor adenocarcinoma" in a small biopsy specimen. Resection specimens allow a more detailed subclassification. There has been significant refinement in adenocarcinoma classification in recent years based on close pathologic and clinical correlation.[3,8] The major histologic types have been validated to bear prognostic significance delineated by the tumor grade.[9–14] Multiple gene alterations can occur in adenocarcinomas, with approved molecular targeted therapy available to improve patient survival (see later disccusion).

Box 1
World Health Organization classification of lung cancer

Adenocarcinoma
    Lepidic adenocarcinoma
    Acinar adenocarcinoma
    Papillary adenocarcinoma
    Micropapillary adenocarcinoma
    Solid adenocarcinoma
    Invasive mucinous adenocarcinoma
    Colloid adenocarcinoma
    Fetal adenocarcinoma
    Enteric adenocarcinoma
    Minimally invasive adenocarcinoma

Squamous cell carcinoma

Neuroendocrine tumors
    Carcinoid tumors
        Typical carcinoid
        Atypical carcinoid
    Small cell carcinoma
    Large cell neuroendocrine carcinoma

Large cell carcinoma

Adenosquamous carcinoma

Pleomorphic carcinoma

Spindle cell carcinoma

Giant cell carcinoma

Carcinosarcoma

Pulmonary blastoma

Other and unclassified carcinomas
    Lymphoepithelioma-like carcinoma
    NUT carcinoma

Salivary gland–type carcinomas
    Mucoepidermoid carcinoma
    Adenoid cystic carcinoma
    Epithelial-myoepithelial carcinoma

Mesenchymal tumors, lymphohistiocytic tumors, tumors of ectopic origin, and metastatic tumors

Adapted from Travis WD, Brambila E, Burke AP, et al. WHO classification of tumours of the lung, pleura, thymus and heart. 4th edition. Lyon (France): IARC Press; 2015.

Preinvasive or Minimally Invasive Adenocarcinoma

Adenocarcinoma in situ (AIS) represents relatively small sized tumors (≤3 cm) with neoplastic cells growing along preexisting alveolar structures (lepidic growth pattern) without evidence of stromal, vascular, or pleural invasion. Lepidic is a descriptive term for rind or membranous growth pattern and is now specifically used to describe tumor cells proliferating along the surface of intact alveolar walls.[15] Lepidic growth usually correlates with ground glass opacity on radiograms. Most AISs are the nonmucinous type, with mild to moderate pleomorphic cuboidal to columnar tumor cells linearly lining alveolar walls. There is no secondary papillary or micropapillary growth pattern. A

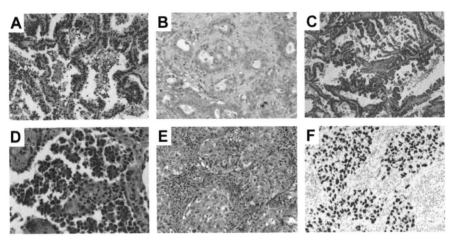

Fig. 1. Adenocarcinomas. (*A*) Lepidic adenocarcinoma (H&E, original magnification ×200). (*B*) Acinar adenocarcinoma (H&E, original magnification ×200). (*C*) Papillary adenocarcinoma (H&E, original magnification ×100). (*D*) Micropapillary adenocarcinoma (H&E, original magnification ×200). (*E*) Solid adenocarcinoma (H&E, original magnification ×100). (*F*) Solid adenocarcinoma (TTF-1 stain, original magnification ×100).

minority of such tumors are of mucinous or mixed type. If the tumor contains a small focus (<5 mm) of invasive growth, the tumor is classified microinvasive adenocarcinoma (MIA). Invasion usually induces formation of a desmoplastic stroma. Invasion can also manifest as nonlepidic growth, such as acinar, papillary, micropapillary, or solid patterns. MIA is defined not only by limited size invasive growth but also by a lack of more advanced invasive pattern, such as tumor necrosis, lymphovascular invasion, and pleural invasion. Both types of tumor are low grade and have a nearly 100% 5-year survival rate.[3]

Invasive Adenocarcinoma

Most invasive adenocarcinomas are composed of mixed morphological subtypes; these are classified according to the predominant architectural structures rather than lumped together as mixed subtype. Each tumor is classified according to one predominant growth pattern, including lepidic, acinar, papillary, micropapillary, and solid patterns (see **Fig. 1**). Each additional subpattern is recorded semiquantitatively as estimated percentage in 5% increments.[3,8] This architectural-driven classification has prognostic significance, with most favorable prognosis for lepidic-predominant adenocarcinomas, intermediate survival rate for acinar and papillary predominant adenocarcinomas, and poor prognosis for solid and micropapillary predominant adenocarcinomas.[11,12,16]

Lepidic Adenocarcinoma

Lepidic growth is commonly seen in lung adenocarcinoma. The lepidic growth pattern denotes tumor cells spreading along preexisting alveolar structures, although there may be sclerotic thickening of alveolar septa. When it is the predominant growth pattern with additional findings that set it apart from previously described AIS and MIA, it is designated as lepidic adenocarcinoma. These additional findings include any one or more of the following: more than 5 mm of invasion (presence of desmoplastic or myofibroblastic stroma); spread through air spaces; lymphatic or vascular invasion; pleural invasion; tumor necrosis. Although such tumors were previously classified as bronchioloalveolar carcinoma, this term is no longer used because it encompasses a heterogeneous group of adenocarcinomas. This category convenes a significantly better prognosis than other subtypes.[3]

Acinar Adenocarcinoma

Acinar adenocarcinoma is a common type of adenocarcinoma with tumor cells arranged in classic glandular structure on a fibroelastic stroma. It is important to separate demosplastic stroma in this pattern from preexisting alveolar structures with thickened fibroelastic alveolar septa sometimes seen in a lepidic pattern. It is of note that the tumor cells displaying more complex growth patterns, such as a cribriform pattern, likely represent a poor prognostic subtype convening a significant risk of recurrence.[17]

Papillary Adenocarcinoma

The tumor cells form papillary architecture with tumor cells lining the surface of branching fibrovascular cores. The presence of fibrovascular cores separates this tumor type from micropapillary adenocarcinoma.

Micropapillary Adenocarcinoma

The tumor cells form individual cellular tufts without fibrovascular core. The tumor cells appear as detached small and solid individual cell groups. Psammoma bodies may be seen. This subtype of adenocarcinoma has distinctly poor prognosis in the early stage compared with other subtypes of adenocarcinoma.[18–20]

Solid Adenocarcinoma

The tumor cells form patternless sheets and lack any other recognizable patterns, including poorly differentiated/undifferentiated carcinomas expressing pneumocytic markers (such as TTF-1 and NapsinA), which were formerly grouped in the LCC category.[3] It is of note that certain markers commonly associated with squamous cell differentiation, such as p63, and less commonly, p40, can show focal expression in solid adenocarcinoma.[3,21]

Rare Variants of Invasive Adenocarcinoma

Rare variants of invasive adenocarcinoma include invasive mucinous adenocarcinoma, colloid and fetal adenocarcinoma, and enteric adenocarcinoma. Invasive mucinous adenocarcinoma is frequently multicentric and the tumor cells lack expression of TTF-1 commonly seen for lung adenocarcinoma.[22] Enteric adenocarcinoma should be distinguished from metastatic colorectal adenocarcinoma.[23]

SQUAMOUS CELL CARCINOMA

SCCs make up about 20% of lung cancers.[4] Their incidence has declined in recent decades, likely because of changes in smoking behavior. SCC usually occurs in the central portion of the lung, along major airways, and can form cavities when it achieves a large size. On microscopic examination, SCC characteristically shows keratinization and intercellular bridges and exhibits a solid nested growth pattern (**Fig. 2**). The tumor cells usually have hyperchromatic nuclei, visible to inconspicuous nucleoli, and moderate to abundant cytoplasm with delineated intercellular bridges. There can be individual tumor cell keratinization or groups of keratinizing squamous cells forming keratin pearls centrally placed within solid tumor nests. The tumor cells lack glandular

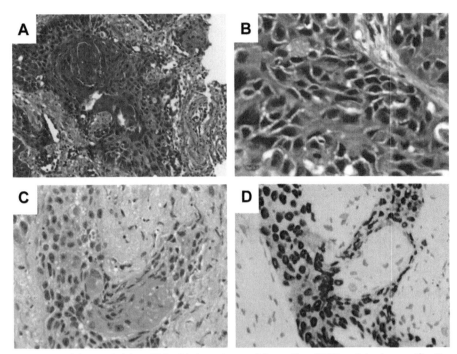

Fig. 2. SCC. (*A*) Keratinizing SCC with keratin pearl formation (H&E, original magnification ×200). (*B*) Intercellular bridge formation (H&E, original magnification ×400). (*C*) Nonkeratinizing SCC without apparent keratinization or discernible intercellular bridges (H&E, original magnification ×400). (*D*) Tumor cells stain positive for p40 (nuclear stain) (p40 stain, original magnification ×400).

structure or mucin production. SCCs are further divided into keratinizing, nonkeratinizing, and basaloid subtypes. Contrary to adenocarcinoma subtypes, such subclassification shows no apparent prognostic utility except for basaloid SCCs, which reportedly display distinct molecular profile conferring intrinsic resistance to cytotoxic chemotherapy.[24] Recognizing morphologic features of squamous cell differentiation, including keratinization, keratin pearl formation, and intercellular bridges, establishes SCC diagnosis, even in small biopsy specimens. When the tumor is poorly differentiated and does not allow confident morphologic classification, selective squamous cell markers, such as p40, CK5/6, CK5, and p63, are used to demonstrate squamous differentiation (see **Fig. 2**).[25] TTF-1 stain is usually negative, although focal weak positive stain for this marker has been reported.[26] Poorly differentiated tumor defined by expression of squamous cell markers in a biopsy material is diagnosed as "NSCC, favor SCC." Although tumors in this category are usually excluded from current molecular testing, identification of driver mutations in SCC, such as discoidin domain receptor 2 (DDR2), phosphatidylinositol-4,5-bisphosphate 3-kinase catalytic subunit alpha (PI3KCA), fibroblastic growth factor receptor 1 (FGFR1), and v-akt murine thymoma viral oncogene homolog 1 (AKT1), may enable future personalized therapy.[27] Establishment of squamous cell differentiation has important implications in chemotherapeutic agent choices so as to avoid certain complications. For instance, treatment with the vascular endothelial growth factor inhibitor bevacizumab in patients with SCC can potentially precipitate life-threatening pulmonary hemorrhage, and therefore, should be avoided.[28,29] Survival rate for SCC is significantly better than adenocarcinoma.

LARGE CELL CARCINOMA

LCCs represent a minority of NSCC cases that are devoid of lineage-specific differentiation, and lack morphologic and immunohistochemical evidence of adenocarcinoma, SCC, or neuroendocrine carcinoma (null immunophenotype). LCC is usually peripherally located, bulky, and necrotic in appearance. The tumor cells are large and polygonal in shape with pleomorphic and vesicular nuclei. The tumor cells form patternless solid sheet or nests. Large cell neuroendocrine carcinoma (LCNEC) is classified in the lung neuroendocrine tumor (NET) category (see later discussion). LCCs represent less than 3% of the lung cancers.[4,23] Tumors with morphologic characteristic of LCC are designated as "NSCC, not otherwise specified (NOS)" in a biopsy or cytology material, not LCC, because the latter can only be ascertained in a resection specimen with the thoroughly analyzed tumor devoid of lineage-specific differentiation.[3,5] It is important to apply ancillary tests such as IHC to avoid inclusion of poorly differentiated NSCC, such as solid adenocarcinoma and nonkeratinizing SCC, in this category. In fact, most LCCs defined by morphologic criteria can be reclassified as adenocarcinoma and SCC using a panel of lineage-specific markers.[30–32] Effective application of such ancillary tests is the likely explanation for the decline of lung cancers categorized as LCC in recent years.[3] Recent evidence suggests that tumors currently classified as LCC with null immunophenotype share molecular characteristics similar to solid adenocarcinoma.[33] Tumors in this category are not necessarily excluded from molecular testing. Metastatic tumors should be excluded in appropriate clinical context. Most LCC cases have adverse outcome, especially for those with null immunophenotype.[34]

OTHER NON–SMALL CELL CARCINOMA TYPES

Adenosquamous carcinoma is a rare type of NSCC, accounting for less than 5% of all lung cancers.[35] It represents a hybrid carcinoma containing both adenocarcinoma and SCC components, with each comprising at least 10% of the tumor.[2,3] From a clinical prospective, adenosquamous carcinoma is usually included in the discussion of adenocarcinomas because therapeutically important mutations occur in adenosquamous carcinoma in similar frequency as in conventional adenocarcinoma[36]; this is especially significant in light of its worse prognosis than that of adenocarcinoma and SCC.[37–39]

Pleomorphic, spindle cell, and giant cell carcinomas are rare types of NSCC, accounting for less than 3% of lung cancers.[3] These tumors demonstrate spindle and/or giant cell differentiation (sarcoma-like differentiation). Such tumors can be ascertained only in resection specimens. In biopsy specimens, tumors with such features are reported as "NSCC with spindle and/or giant cell carcinoma."[3,8] Expression of cytokeratin is important in this setting to exclude a primary pulmonary sarcoma. Because some tumors can show weak or even absent expression of common epithelial markers, multiple anticytokeratin antibodies may be necessary. Epithelial markers commonly used include pancytokeratin, cytokeratin AE1/AE3, CK7, and EMA. Such tumors have a worse prognosis than conventional NSCC.[40]

Carcinosarcoma is composed of NSCC and sarcomatous elements, such as rhabdomyosarcoma, chondrosarcoma, and osteosarcoma.[3] Pulmonary blastoma must be distinguished from pleuropulmonary blastoma occurring in the pediatric population.[41] Carcinomas can rarely arise from bronchial glands, analogous to salivary gland tissue. Major histologic types include mucoepidermoid carcinoma, adenoid cystic carcinoma, and epithelial-myoepithelial carcinoma.[3]

NEUROENDOCRINE TUMORS

NETs as a group are relatively common lung tumors, accounting for about 20% to 25% of lung cancers.[42,43] Their common morphologic, immunohistochemical, and ultrastructural features set them apart from other lung tumors. These features include organoid growth pattern, finely granular or "salt-and-pepper" chromatin pattern, and the expression of several hallmark neuroendocrine markers. Common neuroendocrine markers include chromogranin A, synaptophysin, and CD56. Within this group of tumors, there is a heterogeneous degree of differentiation, with well-differentiated tumors retaining most or all of the above characteristics and poorly differentiated tumors losing some or most of the discernible neuroendocrine differentiation features. This histologic differentiation is epitomized by tumor proliferation rate, which in turn correlates with tumor aggressiveness and prognosis. The 2015 WHO classification separates this group of tumors into 4 major categories, including typical carcinoid, atypical carcinoid, small cell carcinoma (or SCLC), and LCNEC (**Table 1**).[3] Because tumor cell proliferation rate has been shown to provide accurate overall prognostic information, this has been used along with the presence or absence of necrosis to divide NETs into 3 grades of prognostic significance.[44–46] The low-grade NET corresponds to typical carcinoid; intermediate-grade NET corresponds to atypical carcinoid, and high-grade NET corresponds to SCLC and LCNEC. The proliferation rate is expressed as the number of mitoses per microscopic unit area of tumor (usually defined as mitoses per 2 mm^2 or 10 high-magnification microscopic fields). In recent years, utilization of Ki67 labeling index as an adjunct for grading has gained popularity.[47–49] This Ki67 labeling index is especially useful in evaluating small biopsy specimens, whereby it is often impossible to count adequate microscopic fields to give an accurate reflection of proliferation rate.

Typical Carcinoid

Carcinoid tumors are rare, accounting for 1% to 2% of all lung tumors.[48] In the pediatric population, however, carcinoid tumors represent a common tumor type.[50,51]

Table 1
Diagnostic findings in neuroendocrine tumors

	Typical Carcinoid	Atypical Carcinoid	SCLC	LCNEC
Neuroendocrine morphology	Monotonous cells arranged in organoid nesting, palisading, rosettes, trabeculae	Monotonous cells arranged in organoid nesting, palisading, rosettes, trabeculae	Small cell size, finely granular chromatin, inconspicuous nucleoli, scanty cytoplasm	Large cell size, frequent presence of nucleoli, abundant cytoplasm
Mitoses per 2 mm^2	<2	2–10	>10, usually >60	>10, usually >30
Ki67 proliferation index	≤4–5%	≤20–25%	>50%	Usually >40%
Necrosis	No	Focal or punctuate	Often extensively present	Often extensively present
Neuroendocrine marker expression	Yes	Yes	Yes, rarely negative	Yes
Grade	Low grade	Intermediate grade	High grade	High grade

Typical carcinoids are different from other types of lung cancers in their presentation at a relatively younger age (mean age range at presentation 45–55 years) and more frequent presentation at an earlier stage (more than 70% of the cases present as stage I disease), as well as good prognosis (more than 90% 5-year survival rate).[52] There is no direct association with smoking because the prevalence of smoking in patients diagnosed for typical carcinoid is similar to the general population.[53] Carcinoid syndrome is rarely present, unless there is liver metastasis.[54] Carcinoid tumors occur in about 5% of patients with multiple endocrine neoplasia type 1, although most cases occur as nonfamilial (sporadic) isolated tumors.[55]

Typical carcinoids display characteristic morphologic features attributable to neuroendocrine differentiation. The tumor cells are generally small in size and uniform in shape. The chromatin pattern is usually fine or coarse granular without apparent nucleoli. There is a moderate amount of eosinophilic staining cytoplasm, which keeps individual tumor cell nuclei a uniform distance from one another. The tumor cells are typically arranged in organoid nests, with variation of trabeculae, insular, ribbon, and rosettelike arrangements (**Fig. 3**). Some typical carcinoids have spindle cell features with fusiform cells arranged in a fascicular pattern. By definition, typical carcinoids have a low proliferation rate, less than 2 mitoses per 10 high power fields. Ki67 (or MIB-1) labeling index is usually less than 4% to 5%.[49] There is no tumor necrosis. Typical carcinoid expresses common neuroendocrine markers such as synaptophysin, chromogranin, and CD56.

Atypical Carcinoid

Similar to typical carcinoids, atypical carcinoids are relatively common in the younger age group compared with other types of lung cancers and are frequently presented as early-staged disease.[48] The prevalence of smoking in patients diagnosed for atypical carcinoids is twice as high as the general population. The prognosis of atypical

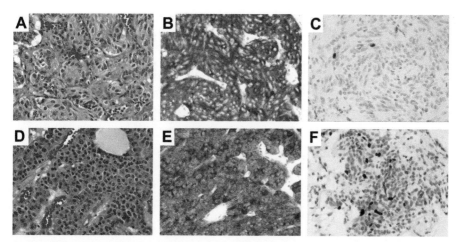

Fig. 3. NETs. (*A*) Typical carcinoid with organoid cell nests (H&E, original magnification ×400). (*B*) Typical carcinoid with positive staining for synaptophysin (synaptophysin stain, original magnification ×400). (*C*) Typical carcinoid with less than 4% Ki67 labeling index (Ki67 stain, original magnification ×400). (*D*) Atypical carcinoid with organoid cell nests (H&E, original magnification ×400). (*E*) Atypical carcinoid with positive staining for synaptophysin (synaptophysin stain, original magnification ×400). (*F*) Atypical carcinoid with greater than 4% Ki67 labeling index (Ki67 stain, original magnification ×400).

carcinoid is significantly lower than typical carcinoid, with 5-year overall survival rate less than 80%.[56]

Atypical carcinoids have cytomorphological features similar to typical carcinoids, although tumor cells in atypical carcinoids tend to display more cytologic atypia (see **Fig. 3**). The defining features of the atypical carcinoids are an intermediate proliferation rate and/or the presence of tumor necrosis. Atypical carcinoids have an intermediate rate of mitosis, between 2 and 10 mitoses per 2 mm².[3] Ki67 or MIB-1 labeling index is usually less than 20% to 25%.[46,49] Evaluation of Ki67 labeling index can be important in a small biopsy material to avoid overdiagnosing atypical carcinoids as high-grade neuroendocrine carcinomas.[47] Tumor necrosis is focally present, usually punctuate, and less than 10% of the tumor volume.[49]

Small Cell Carcinoma

Small cell carcinomas or SCLCs comprise slightly more than 10% of all lung cancers.[4,57] Smoking history is present in virtually all cases of SCLC.[4] SCLC is a highly aggressive malignancy. Patients usually have metastatic disease at the time of presentation. Most patients relapse within the first 2 years after treatment and the 2-year survival rate is less than 10% in metastatic patients.[58] SCLC is commonly centrally located in the major airway. SCLC has distinct morphologic features and careful evaluation on the routine hematoxylin and eosin (H&E)-stained section affords a high accuracy of diagnosis. The tumor cells are small in size compared with other types of lung cancers, usually less than the diameter of 3 mature lymphocytes. The chromatin is finely granular without prominent nucleoli. The cytoplasm is scanty, and the cellular borders are inconspicuous (**Fig. 4**). There is a high mitotic rate, usually greater than 10 mitoses per 2 mm². There is also a high apoptotic rate and frequent presence of

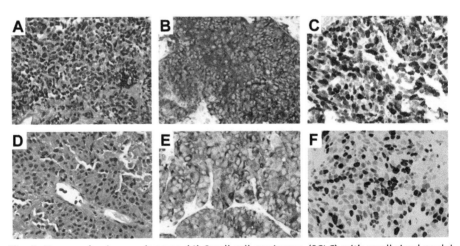

Fig. 4. Neuroendocrine carcinomas. (*A*) Small cell carcinoma (SCLC) with small-sized nuclei and scanty cytoplasm (H&E, original magnification ×400). (*B*) SCLC with positive staining for synaptophysin (synaptophysin stain, original magnification ×400). (*C*) SCLC with greater than 80% Ki67 labeling index (Ki67 stain, original magnification ×400). (*D*) LCNEC with large-sized cells and tumor necrosis (H&E, original magnification ×400). (*E*) LCNEC with positive staining for synaptophysin (synaptophysin stain, original magnification ×400). (*F*) LCNEC with greater than 40% Ki67 labeling index (Ki67 stain, original magnification ×400).

extensive tumor necrosis. In bronchial biopsy material, there is frequent crush artifact. In core needle biopsy or surgical biopsy specimen, there is usually greater nuclear size variation and less crush artifact. The tumor cells form organoid nests or diffuse sheets. The diagnosis is based on light microscopy using routine H&E-stained slides. In small biopsy material with significant crush artifact, IHC can be very helpful in establishing the diagnosis and in excluding other morphologic mimics. Commonly used stains include pankeratin and neuroendocrine markers (CD56, chromogranin, synaptophysin), although their expression levels are usually lower than low- to intermediate-grade NETs. An exception is TTF-1, which is expressed in close to 90% of SCLC.[59,60] High Ki67 (MIB-1) labeling index (>50%, usually 70%–100%) is a hallmark of SCLC, which helps to distinguish it from low- and intermediate-grade NETs to avoid overdiagnosing the latter in small crushed biopsy specimens.[47,49] Cytology is extremely useful and can offer a higher yield of diagnosis than small biopsies with scant intact, viable tumor cells. WHO classification divides SCLC into 2 subtypes: pure SCLC and combined SCLC containing a component of NSCC.

Large Cell Neuroendocrine Carcinoma

LCNEC, like SCLC, is associated with heavy smoking history.[4] It is usually peripherally located in the lung. LCNEC is a highly aggressive neuroendocrine carcinoma. As its name implies, the tumor cells are larger than SCLCs and they have abundant cytoplasm (see **Fig. 4**). Other common features include polygonal cell shape, frequent presence of nucleoli, and low nuclear-cytoplasmic (N:C) ratio.[61] Importantly, there is discernible neuroendocrine architecture, including organoid arrangement, trabecular growth, and rosettelike structures. There is a noticeable absence of cellular architectures commonly associated with adenocarcinoma differentiation. Like SCLC, these tumors show high mitotic rate (>10 mitoses per 2 mm^2) and conspicuous tumor necrosis. Immunohistochemical stains play an important ancillary role. There should be expression of at least one neuroendocrine marker. It is of note that the diagnosis of LCNEC is based on a combination of the above features. Specifically, the diagnosis is not relied solely on immunohistochemical expression of neuroendocrine markers because up to 20% of NSCCs (adenocarcinoma, SCC, and LCC) show demonstrable positive immunohistochemical staining for neuroendocrine markers.[2,22] Such tumors are classified as their NSCC type with neuroendocrine differentiation. Combined LCNEC has components of other types of NSCC or SCLC. LCNEC is a highly aggressive tumor, and 5-year survival rate is reported close to 30%, significantly worse than other types of NSCC.[62]

OTHER PRIMARY TUMORS OF THE LUNG

Besides lung carcinomas as described above, other types of tumors can arise from lung, including mesenchymal tumors, lymphohistiocytic tumors, melanoma, germ cell tumors, and others.[3]

BIOPSY DIAGNOSIS OF LUNG CANCER

Lung cancer diagnosis and classification provide pivotal information for prognosis and guide selection of therapeutic regimens. Most lung cancers are presented in advanced stage, requiring tissue biopsy or cytology diagnosis. The purpose of tissue biopsy includes establishment of malignancy diagnosis based on histomorphological findings, classification of tumor type and grade aided by IHC staining, and obtaining cellular material for targeted therapy-driven molecular testing. To minimize the occurrence of nondiagnostic or repeat biopsies, a multidisciplinary approach with input from pathology, radiology, pulmonology, surgery, and oncology teams is warranted, with effective tissue sampling strategy preferably established in prospective tumor board case discussion.[25] To maximize the probability of productive biopsy workup, biopsy samples should be prioritized for the following three key steps of analysis: The first step is morphologic evaluation using H&E-stained slides. Diagnosis of better differentiated NSCC can be established based on the presence of glandular structure and/or mucin production (adenocarcinoma) or apparent formation of keratinization and intercellular bridges (SCC). Less well-differentiated NSCC and NET (including SCLC) usually require a second step of IHC confirmation. Concise IHC panel should be selected, guided by morphologic analysis. An effective way to accomplish both steps while preserving tissue material is to precut blank slides for potential IHC stains at the time of initial tissue sectioning for H&E stain. Such strategy minimizes the need to put the tissue block back to the microtome, shortens the diagnosis turn-around time, and maximizes the amount of tissue preserved in the tissue block for the third step of molecular biomarker testing.[25,63] Efficient triage and utilization of small biopsy specimens for molecular testing require effective communication and coordinated effort of a multidisciplinary team to complete an appropriate testing menu.

IMMUNOHISTOCHEMISTRY

The most important ancillary method in lung cancer diagnosis and classification is IHC. IHC stains are performed on tissue slides and can be readily integrated into laboratory diagnostic practice. The significance of applying IHC includes aiding effective and accurate classification of tumors (especially for poorly differentiated tumors in small biopsy specimens), minimizing potential diagnostic errors, improving delineation of tumor types suitable for molecular testing, and utilizing lineage-specific markers for the exclusion of metastatic origin of the tumors. IHC markers are most effective if appropriate markers are judiciously selected and used as a panel. There is significant recent progress in cataloging of the biomarkers, and application of IHC has been emphasized in the current WHO classification.[3] One of the most important applications of IHC is to separate adenocarcinomas from SCC. When these tumors are poorly differentiated, an accurate distinction between the two usually requires IHC analysis, even for resected specimens.[64] In certain instances, IHC provides a more accurate tumor classification because in rare occasions adenocarcinomas can have a solid or pseudosquamous morphology.[65,66] Commonly used markers to ascertain adenocarcinoma differentiation include TTF-1 and NapsinA, expressed in more than 85% of the adenocarcinomas.[6,7,63] Expression of either of these two markers is considered de facto evidence of adenocarcinoma or adenocarcinoma differentiation in NSCC if other tumors that also commonly express these markers (including SCLC and LCNEC) can be excluded. IHC markers commonly expressed in SCC include p40, CK5/6, CK5, and p63 (**Table 2**). A tumor can be considered SCC if any of these markers are expressed in the absence of adenocarcinoma-specific marker expression. One exception is p63, which is less specific than the other markers because it can also be expressed in close to 20% of adenocarcinomas.[21] Using these stains, about 90% of the poorly differentiated NSCC can be classified as either adenocarcinoma or SCC.[65,67] A poorly differentiated carcinoma that is negative for all the above markers (null immunophenotype) can be classified as "NSCC, NOS" in a biopsy specimen.[5] An effective way to achieve diagnostic accuracy while conserving biopsy material is to use antibody cocktails or double labeling.[6,7,68]

Table 2
Differential immunohistochemical characteristics of adenocarcinoma and squamous cell carcinoma

Antibody	Adenocarcinoma	SCC
TTF-1	+	−
NapsinA	+	−
P40	−	+
CK5/6	−	+
CK5	−	+
P63	−	+
Desmoglein-3	−	+

Abbreviation: CK, cytokeratin.

A second effective utilization of IHC is to reclassify or identify adenocarcinoma and SCC differentiation in LCC. Using a panel of IHC, most morphologically diagnosed LCC can be accurately reclassified as adenocarcinoma or SCC.[30,31] Cytokeratin markers are important in diagnosing pleomorphic, spindle cell, and giant cell carcinomas. Multiple epithelial markers, such as pancytokeratin, cytokeratin AE1/3, CK7, and EMA, may be necessary to confirm epithelial differentiation and to exclude pulmonary sarcomas.

IHC is also useful in demonstrating neuroendocrine differentiation in tumors exhibiting neuroendocrine morphology. Commonly used neuroendocrine markers include CD56, synaptophysin, and chromogranin. NETs also express other markers commonly used in a panel IHC workup, including cytokeratins, CK7, TTF-1, NapsinA, and p63. An IHC panel for the confirmation of SCLC diagnosis includes pankeratin (usually dotlike perinuclear staining), neuroendocrine markers (CD56, chromogranin, and synaptophysin), TTF-1 (70%–90% positivity), and Ki67 (70%–100% labeling index).

As a surrogate test for molecular profiling of NSCC (see later discussion), IHC has been evaluated as a rapid and cost-effective testing platform deployable in the routine pathology practice setting in the determination of predictive biomarkers. Several mutation-specific antibodies have been developed. For instance, epidermal growth factor (EGFR) mutation-specific antibodies demonstrate a good specificity, albeit with limited sensitivity.[69,70] In comparison, the sensitivity and specificity of antibodies against anaplastic lymphoma kinase (ALK) and C-ros oncogene 1 (ROS1) are more consistent. Several monoclonal antibodies recognizing ALK protein have shown promising results to screen for ALK gene rearrangement comparable to fluorescence in situ hybridization (FISH) method.[71–73] IHC using an antibody specific for ROS1 protein has achieved high specificity and sensitivity in detecting ROS1-translocated tumors and can act as an effective screening tool.[74]

Lung is a frequent target of metastasis, and metastatic malignancy to lung is more often encountered in clinical practice than primary lung cancer. Although lung metastasis is often multifocal, it can be solitary. Certain lung cancers can also present as multifocal disease. In this regard, IHC plays a pivotal role in separating primary lung cancer from metastasis. IHC can help confirm the presence of metastasis and identify primary tumor tissue of origin in most cases. A 3-tiered approach helps to separate metastasis from lung cancer. Metastatic tumors usually show distinct CK7 and CK20 expression pattern, absence of markers commonly expressed in primary lung cancers (such as TTF-1 and NapsinA), and expression of organ-associated markers.[75,76]

MOLECULAR TESTING OF LUNG CANCER

Molecular analysis of lung cancer genetic alterations has both advanced the understanding of carcinogenesis and provided a paradigm change in therapeutic targeting and monitoring. Detection of specific genetic alterations has been proved to be effective in predicting treatment response and stratifying prognosis and is potentially applicable in early detection of lung cancer.[77,78] Targeted therapy using drugs specifically designed to inhibit mutation-driven genetic alterations affords more effectiveness and less toxicity than generic chemotherapeutic agents and therefore substantial improvement of outcomes compared with standard chemotherapy in the treatment of advanced NSCC. One of the common mechanisms of carcinogenesis is constitutive activation of receptor tyrosine kinases, such that inhibition of their activity creates an effective modality for anticancer therapy. With the advent of tyrosine kinase inhibitor (TKI) treatments, it is important to screen patients with lung cancer for actionable gene mutations. EGFR mutation and ALK translocation are the most effectively targeted oncogenes in NSCC and are now considered standard of care.[79] Recent advancement in testing methodologies such as next-generation sequencing (NGS) affords multiplex systems to detect multiple gene alterations on one single platform.[80] Noninvasive plasma and serum-based DNA detection and monitoring are emerging molecular tools.[81]

EGFR is a transmembrane glycoprotein receptor. Upon ligand binding, activation of its cytoplasmic tyrosine kinase domain by dimerization and phosphorylation elicits downstream signaling pathways that lead to DNA synthesis and cell proliferation. EGFR gain of function mutations lead to constitutive activation of downstream signaling pathways, which is critical for tumor growth.[82,83] EGFR mutations can be detected in 10% to 30% of NSCC patients. Tyrosine phosphorylation inhibitors or TKIs inhibit EGFR phosphorylation and thus are able to mute the effect of EGFR mutations. Hence, detection of EGFR mutations predicts response to targeted therapy using TKIs. As first-line treatment, TKIs have been shown to produce overall response rates of close to 75% in tumors carrying EGFR mutations.[84] Because EGFR mutations are detected mostly in adenocarcinomas, the current recommendation is to test for EGFR mutations in adenocarcinomas, mixed lung cancers with an adenocarcinoma component (such as adenosquamous carcinoma), and small samples whereby an adenocarcinoma component cannot be excluded.[79] Molecular biological techniques for EGFR mutation detection include screening methods that detect all mutations and targeted methods that detect specific, known types of mutations. Commonly used screening methods include direct DNA sequencing and high-resolution melting analysis. Targeted methods include polymerase chain reaction (PCR) -based targeted methods, such as ARMS (Amplification Refractory Mutation SystemARMS) and SmartAMP (Smart Amplification Process).[85,86] Gefitinib, erlotinib, and afatinib are currently recommended TKIs for first-line treatment of those with sensitizing EGFR mutations in lung cancer.[87–89] Development of an additional mutation T790M is a common mechanism for acquired resistance to TKI treatment. Possible strategies to overcome such acquired drug resistance include platinum-based doublet chemotherapy and utilization of next-generation PKIs.[90]

ALK is another receptor tyrosine kinase. A common form of ALK alteration is the formation of an oncogenic fusion gene with echinoderm microtubule-associated protein-like 4 (EML4-ALK), seen in 4% to 7% of NSCCs, particularly adenocarcinomas.[91]

Thus, ALK testing is similarly recommended for adenocarcinomas and mixed lung cancers with an adenocarcinoma component.[79] ALK gene rearrangements are found to be mutually exclusive with EGFR and KRAS mutations.[92] Commonly used molecular methods for detecting EML4-ALK fusion gene include real-time PCR, FISH, and direct DNA sequencing.[86,93] The ALK competitive binding inhibitor crizotinib is approved for those with ALK gene rearrangement.[90] In contrast to acquired resistance in EGFR TKI therapy, multiple acquired mutations may develop, resulting in drug resistance. Next-generation ALK TKIs may be a promising treatment approach in crizotinib-resistant cases.[90]

Besides EGFR and ALK, a multitude of other biomarkers are being actively evaluated or used as therapeutic targets.[94] ROS1 is a receptor tyrosine kinase that can be rearranged in 1% to 2% of lung adenocarcinomas. ROS1 rearrangement is rarely found coexisting with EGFR and ALK alterations.[92] Crizotinib has been shown to be effective in patients with ROS1 rearrangement and is approved for such treatment.[95] The mesenchymal epithelial transition factor (MET) gene is also a transmembrane tyrosine kinase receptor that can be altered by either overexpression or amplification. Such genetic alterations have been shown to be an adverse prognostic marker.[96] MET amplification is also a common mechanism for acquired resistance to EGFR TKI therapy.[97] Therapeutic coinhibition of both receptors may represent a potential treatment option to overcome such acquired drug resistance. Kirsten rat sarcoma viral oncogene homolog (KRAS) belongs to the RAS family of oncogenes together with HRAS and NRAS. The KRAS gene encodes a GTP-binding protein. Mutations in KRAS are usually mutually exclusive with other oncogenic driver mutations.[98] Development of KRAS inhibitor is still ongoing, and a phase III trial of the downstream RAS pathway inhibitor, selumetinib, has been initiated.[99] Another RAS pathway protein kinase, BRAF, is also a potential target for inhibitor therapy. BRAF mutation occurs in 2% to 3% of NSCC, and V600E is the most common mutation.[94] Other biomarkers under active evaluation include human epidermal growth factor receptor 2, rearranged during transfection, fibroblast growth factor receptor 1 (FGFR1), discoidin domain receptor tyrosine kinase 2 (DDR2), phosphatase and tensin homolog, MAP2K (mitogen-activated protein kinase kinase), and phosphatidylinositol 3 kinase.[94]

Molecular techniques for detecting genomic alterations in lung cancer include screening (or scanning) genotyping methods and targeted genotyping methods. Commonly used screening technologies include Sanger sequencing, pyrosequencing, and high-resolution melt analysis.[100] Targeted assays are designed to detect specific known mutations or "hot-spot" mutations, which afford greater sensitivity. Commonly used targeted assays include Agena MassARRAY Oncocarta panel and SNaPShot multiplex kit.[100] With the necessity to detect an increasing number of gene mutations using often limited biopsy material obtained by minimally invasive procedures, high-efficiency screening and targeted assays have been developed. An ideal detection system should provide adequate sensitivity and specificity in evaluating all clinically relevant genetic alterations in a cost-effective way using a limited sample. This detection system necessitates the implementation of simultaneous evaluation of multiple genes, moving from detecting individual mutations to multiple gene evaluation, or single-tube multiplexed mutation detection. NGS offers a cost-effective approach for detecting multiple genetic alterations with a minimum amount of DNA. NGS provides high-throughput simultaneous sequencing of thousands to millions of short nucleic acid chains in a massively parallel way.[101,102] In targeted NGS, an extended panel of mutations can be screened, covering important mutational hot spots in clinical laboratories.[103,104] NGS can also be used to analyze circulating tumor cells (CTCs) that are shed into the bloodstream from the primary tumor site or metastatic deposit. Tumor cells also release genetic materials in circulation as cell-free circulating tumor DNA (ctDNA) that can be the target for NGS analysis.[105] Such noninvasive "liquid biopsies" conveniently use peripheral blood to provide a surrogate for direct analysis of solid tumors.[106,107] Genetic profiling of CTCs and ctDNA can be used as a proxy parameter for the detection of mutations, evaluation of tumor burden, monitoring of treatment response, and detection of mutation-based treatment resistance, and as a potential tool for screening and early detection of malignancies.

SUMMARY

Classification and histologic typing of lung cancers, together with tumor molecular profiling, lay the foundation on which the oncologic treatment plan is formulated. Since the publication of the last volume, significant update in lung cancer classification has occurred, especially for the subtyping of adenocarcinomas, based on current understanding of tumor biology. This updating is reflected in streamlined classification for small biopsies and cytology specimens, with an emphasis on separating adenocarcinomas from the rest of the lung cancers in order to select tumors for biomarker testing. More detailed histologic typing is used in resection specimens to delineate tissue types of prognostic significance. Immunohistochemistry is an important ancillary method in lung cancer diagnosis and classification. This article seeks to update readers to the new 2015 WHO classification, which delineates major types of lung cancers as adeno-carcinoma, SCC, and NETs. NETs are in turn subdivided into typical carcinoid, atypical carcinoid, small cell carcinoma, and LCNEC based on tumor cell morphology and proliferation rate. Effective application of the recently refined lung cancer classification provides pathologic information fundamental for tumor risk assessment and management decision-making. Molecular profiling has growing importance in identifying subsets of lung cancer with unique sensitivity to targeted therapy.

REFERENCES

1. Pao W, Girard N. New driver mutations in non-small-cell lung cancer. Lancet Oncol 2011;12(2):175–80.
2. Travis WD, Brambilla E, Müller-Hermelink HK, et al. Pathology and genetics of tumours of the lung, pleura, thymus and heart. World Health Organization classification of tumours, series 7. Lyon (France): IARC Press; 2004.
3. Travis WD, Brambila E, Burke AP, et al. WHO classification of tumours of the lung, pleura, thymus and heart. 4th edition. Lyon (France): IARC Press; 2015.
4. Lewis DR, Check DP, Caporaso NE, et al. US lung cancer trends by histologic type. Cancer 2014;120(18):2883–92.
5. Mukhopadhyay S, Katzenstein AL. Subclassification of non-small cell lung carcinomas lacking morphologic differentiation on biopsy specimens: utility of an immunohistochemical panel containing TTF-1, napsin A, p63, and CK5/6. Am J Surg Pathol 2011;35(1):15–25.
6. Rekhtman N, Ang DC, Sima CS, et al. Immunohistochemical algorithm for differentiation of lung adenocarcinoma and squamous cell carcinoma based on large series of whole-tissue sections with validation in small specimens. Mod Pathol 2011;24(10):1348–59.
7. Tacha D, Yu C, Bremer R, et al. A 6-antibody panel for the classification of lung adenocarcinoma versus squamous cell carcinoma. Appl Immunohistochem Mol Morphol 2012;20(3):201–7.
8. Travis WD, Brambilla E, Noguchi M, et al. International Association for the Study of Lung Cancer/American Thoracic Society/European Respiratory Society

international multidisciplinary classification of lung adenocarcinoma. J Thorac Oncol 2011;6(2):244–85.

9. Sica G, Yoshizawa A, Sima CS, et al. A grading system of lung adenocarcinomas based on histologic pattern is predictive of disease recurrence in stage I tumors. Am J Surg Pathol 2010;34(8):1155–62.

10. Russell PA, Wainer Z, Wright GM, et al. Does lung adenocarcinoma subtype predict patient survival?: a clinicopathologic study based on the new International Association for the Study of Lung Cancer/American Thoracic Society/European Respiratory Society international multidisciplinary lung adenocarcinoma classification. J Thorac Oncol 2011;6(9):1496–504.

11. Yoshizawa A, Motoi N, Riely GJ, et al. Impact of proposed IASLC/ATS/ERS classification of lung adenocarcinoma: prognostic subgroups and implications for further revision of staging based on analysis of 514 stage I cases. Mod Pathol 2011;24(5):653–64.

12. Yanagawa N, Shiono S, Abiko M, et al. New IASLC/ATS/ERS classification and invasive tumor size are predictive of disease recurrence in stage I lung adenocarcinoma. J Thorac Oncol 2013;8(5):612–8.

13. Tsuta K, Kawago M, Inoue E, et al. The utility of the proposed IASLC/ATS/ERS lung adenocarcinoma subtypes for disease prognosis and correlation of driver gene alterations. Lung Cancer 2013;81(3):371–6.

14. Lee MC, Kadota K, Buitrago D, et al. Implementing the new IASLC/ATS/ERS classification of lung adenocarcinomas: results from international and Chinese cohorts. J Thorac Dis 2014;6(Suppl 5):S568–80.

15. Jones KD. Whence lepidic? The history of a Canadian neologism. Arch Pathol Lab Med 2013;137:1822–4.

16. Woo T, Okudela K, Mitsui H, et al. Prognostic value of the IASLC/ATS/ERS classification of lung adenocarcinoma in stage I disease of Japanese cases. Pathol Int 2012;62(12):785–91.

17. Kadota K, Yeh YC, Sima CS, et al. The cribriform pattern identifies a subset of acinar predominant tumors with poor prognosis in patients with stage I lung adenocarcinoma: a conceptual proposal to classify cribriform predominant tumors as a distinct histologic subtype. Mod Pathol 2014;27(5):690–700.

18. Miyoshi T, Satoh Y, Okumura S, et al. Early-stage lung adenocarcinomas with a micropapillary pattern, a distinct pathologic marker for a significantly poor prognosis. Am J Surg Pathol 2003;27(1):101–9.

19. Tsutsumida H, Nomoto M, Goto M, et al. A micropapillary pattern is predictive of a poor prognosis in lung adenocarcinoma, and reduced surfactant apoprotein A expression in the micropapillary pattern is an excellent indicator of a poor prognosis. Mod Pathol 2007;20(6):638–47.

20. Nitadori J, Bograd AJ, Kadota K, et al. Impact of micropapillary histologic subtype in selecting limited resection vs lobectomy for lung adenocarcinoma of 2cm or smaller. J Natl Cancer Inst 2013;105(16):1212–20.

21. Nonaka D. A study of ΔNp63 expression in lung non-small cell carcinomas. Am J Surg Pathol 2012;36(6):895–9.

22. Travis WD. Pathology of lung cancer. Clin Chest Med 2011;32(4):669–92.

23. Travis WD, Brambilla E, Noguchi M, et al. Diagnosis of lung adenocarcinoma in resected specimens: implications of the 2011 International Association for the Study of Lung Cancer/American Thoracic Society/European Respiratory Society classification. Arch Pathol Lab Med 2013;137(5):685–705.

24. Brambilla C, Laffaire J, Lantuejoul S, et al. Lung squamous cell carcinomas with basaloid histology represent a specific molecular entity. Clin Cancer Res 2014; 20(22):5777–86.
25. Conde E, Angulo B, Izquierdo E, et al. Lung adenocarcinoma in the era of targeted therapies: histological classification, sample prioritization, and predictive biomarkers. Clin Transl Oncol 2013;15(7):503–8.
26. Hayashi T, Sano H, Egashira R, et al. Difference of morphology and immunophenotype between central and peripheral squamous cell carcinomas of the lung. Biomed Res Int 2013;2013:157838.
27. Gold KA, Wistuba II, Kim ES. New strategies in squamous cell carcinoma of the lung: identification of tumor drivers to personalize therapy. Clin Cancer Res 2012;18(11):3002–7.
28. Johnson DH, Fehrenbacher L, Novotny WF, et al. Randomized phase II trial comparing bevacizumab plus carboplatin and paclitaxel with carboplatin and paclitaxel alone in previously untreated locally advanced or metastatic non-small-cell lung cancer. J Clin Oncol 2004;22(11):2184–91.
29. Sandler A, Gray R, Perry MC, et al. Paclitaxel-carboplatin alone or with bevacizumab for non-small-cell lung cancer. N Engl J Med 2006;355(24):2542–50.
30. Pardo J, Martinez-Penuela AM, Sola JJ, et al. Large cell carcinoma of the lung: an endangered species? Appl Immunohistochem Mol Morphol 2009;17(5): 383–92.
31. Barbareschi M, Cantaloni C, Del Vescovo V, et al. Heterogeneity of large cell carcinoma of the lung: an immunophenotypic and miRNA-based analysis. Am J Clin Pathol 2011;136(5):773–82.
32. Sholl LM. Large-cell carcinoma of the lung: a diagnostic category redefined by immunohistochemistry and genomics. Curr Opin Pulm Med 2014;20(4):324–31.
33. Hwang DH, Szeto DP, Perry AS, et al. Pulmonary large cell carcinoma lacking squamous differentiation is clinicopathologically indistinguishable from solid-subtype adenocarcinoma. Arch Pathol Lab Med 2014;138(5):626–35.
34. Rekhtman N, Tafe LJ, Chaft JE, et al. Distinct profile of driver mutations and clinical features in immunomarker-defined subsets of pulmonary large-cell carcinoma. Mod Pathol 2013;26(4):511–22.
35. Fitzgibbons PL, Kern WH. Adenosquamous carcinoma of the lung: a clinical and pathologic study of seven cases. Hum Pathol 1985;16(5):463–6.
36. Tochigi N, Dacic S, Nikiforova M, et al. Adenosquamous carcinoma of the lung: a microdissection study of KRAS and EGFR mutational and amplification status in a western patient population. Am J Clin Pathol 2011;135(5):783–9.
37. Hofmann HS, Knolle J, Neef H. The adenosquamous lung carcinoma: clinical and pathological characteristics. J Cardiovasc Surg (Torino) 1994;35(6):543–7.
38. Maeda H, Matsumura A, Kawabata T, et al. Adenosquamous carcinoma of the lung: surgical results as compared with squamous cell and adenocarcinoma cases. Eur J Cardiothorac Surg 2012;41(2):357–61.
39. Mordant P, Grand B, Cazes A, et al. Adenosquamous carcinoma of the lung: surgical management, pathologic characteristics, and prognostic implications. Ann Thorac Surg 2013;95(4):1189–95.
40. Martin LW, Correa AM, Ordonez NG, et al. Sarcomatoid carcinoma of the lung: a predictor of poor prognosis. Ann Thorac Surg 2007;84(3):973–80.
41. Travis WD. Sarcomatoid neoplasms of the lung and pleura. Arch Pathol Lab Med 2010;134(11):1645–58.
42. Gustafsson BI, Kidd M, Chan A, et al. Bronchopulmonary neuroendocrine tumors. Cancer 2008;113(1):5–21.

43. Litzky LA. Pulmonary neuroendocrine tumors. Surg Pathol 2010;3:27–59.
44. Moran CA, Suster S, Coppola D, et al. Neuroendocrine carcinomas of the lung: a critical analysis. Am J Clin Pathol 2009;131:206–21.
45. Klimstra DS, Modlin IR, Coppola D, et al. The pathologic classification of neuroendocrine tumors: a review of nomenclature, grading, and staging systems. Pancreas 2010;39(6):707–12.
46. Rindi G, Klersy C, Inzani F, et al. Grading the neuroendocrine tumors of the lung: an evidence-based proposal. Endocr Relat Cancer 2014;21(1):1–16.
47. Lin O, Olgac S, Green I, et al. Immunohistochemical staining of cytologic smears with MIB-1 helps distinguish low-grade from high-grade neuroendocrine neoplasms. Am J Clin Pathol 2003;120(2):209–16.
48. Pelosi G, Rodriguez J, Viale G, et al. Typical and atypical pulmonary carcinoid tumor overdiagnosed as small-cell carcinoma on biopsy specimens: a major pitfall in the management of lung cancer patients. Am J Surg Pathol 2005; 29(2):179–87.
49. Rekhtman N. Neuroendocrine tumors of the lung: an update. Arch Pathol Lab Med 2010;134(11):1628–38.
50. Dishop MK, Kuruvilla S. Primary and metastatic lung tumors in the pediatric population: a review and 25-year experience at a large children's hospital. Arch Pathol Lab Med 2008;132(7):1079–103.
51. Yu DC, Grabowski MJ, Kozakewich HP, et al. Primary lung tumors in children and adolescents: a 90-year experience. J Pediatr Surg 2010;45(6):1090–5.
52. Filosso PL, Guerrera F, Evangelista A, et al. Prognostic model of survival for typical bronchial carcinoid tumours: analysis of 1109 patients on behalf of the European Society of Thoracic Surgeons (ESTS) Neuroendocrine Tumours Working Group. Eur J Cardiothorac Surg 2015;48(3):441–7.
53. Fink G, Krelbaum T, Yellin A, et al. Pulmonary carcinoid: presentation, diagnosis, and outcome in 142 cases in Israel and review of 640 cases from the literature. Chest 2001;119(6):1647–51.
54. Hoberock TR, Knutson CO, Polk HC Jr. Clinical aspects of invasive carcinoid tumors. South Med J 1975;68(1):33–7.
55. Sachithanandan N, Harle RA, Burgess JR. Bronchopulmonary carcinoid in multiple endocrine neoplasia type 1. Cancer 2005;103(3):509–15.
56. Filosso PL, Rena O, Guerrera F, et al. Clinical management of atypical carcinoid and large-cell neuroendocrine carcinoma: a multicentre study on behalf of the European Society of Thoracic Surgeons (ESTS) Neuroendocrine Tumours of the Lung Working Group. Eur J Cardiothorac Surg 2015;48(1):55–64.
57. National Cancer Institute. Surveillance, Epidemiology, and End Results (SEER) Cancer Statistics Review 1975-2010. Available at: http://seer.concer.gov/csr/1975_2010/. Accessed January 15, 2016.
58. Planchard D, Le Pechoux C. Small cell lung cancer: new clinical recommendations and current status of biomarker assessment. Eur J Cancer 2011;47(Suppl 3):S272–83.
59. Nakamura N, Miyagi E, Murata S, et al. Expression of thyroid transcription factor-1 in normal and neoplastic lung tissues. Mod Pathol 2002;15(10):1058–67.
60. Zamecnik J, Kodet R. Value of thyroid transcription factor-1 and surfactant apoprotein A in the differential diagnosis of pulmonary carcinomas: a study of 109 cases. Virchows Arch 2002;440(4):353–61.
61. Travis WD, Linnoila RI, Tsokos MG, et al. Neuroendocrine tumors of the lung with proposed criteria for large-cell neuroendocrine carcinoma. An ultrastructural,

immunohistochemical, and flow cytometric study of 35 cases. Am J Surg Pathol 1991;15(6):529–53.

62. Battafarano RJ, Fernandez FG, Ritter J, et al. Large cell neuroendocrine carcinoma: an aggressive form of non-small cell lung cancer. J Thorac Cardiovasc Surg 2005;130(1):166–72.

63. Mukhopadhyay S. Utility of small biopsies for diagnosis of lung nodules: doing more with less. Mod Pathol 2012;25:S43–57.

64. Kadota K, Nitadori JI, Rekhtman N, et al. Reevaluation and reclassification of resected lung carcinomas originally diagnosed as squamous cell carcinoma using immunohistochemical analysis. Am J Surg Pathol 2015;39(9):1170–80.

65. Pelosi G, Fabbri A, Bianchi F, et al. ΔNp63 (p40) and thyroid transcription factor-1 immunoreactivity on small biopsies or cellblocks for typing non-small cell lung cancer: a novel two-hit, sparing-material approach. J Thorac Oncol 2012;7(2): 281–90.

66. Thunnissen E, Noguchi M, Aisner S, et al. Reproducibility of histopathological diagnosis in poorly differentiated NSCLC: an international multiobserver study. J Thorac Oncol 2014;9(9):1354–62.

67. Loo PS, Thomas SC, Nicolson MC, et al. Subtyping of undifferentiated non-small cell carcinomas in bronchial biopsy specimens. J Thorac Oncol 2010;5(4): 442–7.

68. Brown AF, Sirohi D, Fukuoka J, et al. Tissue-preserving antibody cocktails to differentiate primary squamous cell carcinoma, adenocarcinoma, and small cell carcinoma of lung. Arch Pathol Lab Med 2013;137(9):1274–81.

69. Hasanovic A, Ang D, Moreira AL, et al. Use of mutation specific antibodies to detect EGFR status in small biopsy and cytology specimens of lung adenocarcinoma. Lung Cancer 2012;77(2):299–305.

70. Seo AN, Park TI, Jin Y, et al. Novel EGFR mutation-specific antibodies for lung adenocarcinoma: highly specific but not sensitive detection of an E746_A750 deletion in exon 19 and an L858R mutation in exon 21 by immunohistochemistry. Lung Cancer 2014;83(3):316–23.

71. Mino-Kenudson M, Chirieac LR, Law K, et al. A novel, highly sensitive antibody allows for the routine detection of ALK-rearranged lung adenocarcinomas by standard immunohistochemistry. Clin Cancer Res 2010;16(5):1561–71.

72. Li Y, Pan Y, Wang R, et al. ALK-rearranged lung cancer in Chinese: a comprehensive assessment of clinicopathology, IHC, FISH and RT-PCR. PLoS One 2013;8(7):e69016.

73. Gruber K, Kohlhaufl M, Friedel G, et al. A novel, highly sensitive ALK antibody 1A4 facilitates effective screening for ALK rearrangements in lung adenocarcinomas by standard immunohistochemistry. J Thorac Oncol 2015;10(4):713–6.

74. Sholl LM, Sun H, Butaney M, et al. ROS1 immunohistochemistry for detection of ROS1-rearranged lung adenocarcinomas. Am J Surg Pathol 2013;37(9):1441–9.

75. Lin F, Liu H. Immunohistochemistry in undifferentiated neoplasm/tumor of uncertain origin. Arch Pathol Lab Med 2014;138(12):1583–610.

76. Zhang K, Deng H, Cagle PT. Utility of immunohistochemistry in the diagnosis of pleuropulmonary and mediastinal cancers: a review and update. Arch Pathol Lab Med 2014;138(12):1611–28.

77. Thunnissen E, van der Oord K, den Bakker M. Prognostic and predictive biomarkers in lung cancer. A review. Virchows Arch 2014;464(3):347–58.

78. Verma M. The role of epigenomics in the study of cancer biomarkers and in the development of diagnostic tools. Adv Exp Med Biol 2015;867:59–80.

79. Lindeman NI, Cagle PT, Beasley MB, et al. Molecular testing guideline for selection of lung cancer patients for EGFR and ALK tyrosine kinase inhibitors. Arch Pathol Lab Med 2013;137:828–60.

80. Koboldt DC, Steinberg KM, Larson DE, et al. The next-generation sequencing revolution and its impact on genomics. Cell 2013;155(1):27–38.

81. Nie K, Jia Y, Zhang X. Cell-free circulating tumor DNA in plasma/serum of non-small cell lung cancer. Tumour Biol 2015;36(1):7–19.

82. Linardou H, Dahabreh IJ, Bafaloukos D, et al. Somatic EGFR mutations and efficacy of tyrosine kinase inhibitors in NSCLC. Nat Rev Clin Oncol 2009;6(6): 352–66.

83. Pines G, Köstler WJ, Yarden Y. Oncogenic mutant forms of EGFR: lessons in signal transduction and targets for cancer therapy. FEBS Lett 2010;584(12): 2699–706.

84. Maemondo M, Inoue A, Kobayashi K, et al. Gefitinib or chemotherapy for non-small-cell lung cancer with mutated EGFR. N Engl J Med 2010;362(25):2380–8.

85. Ellison G, Zhu G, Moulis A, et al. EGFR mutation testing in lung cancer: a review of available methods and their use for analysis of tumour tissue and cytology samples. J Clin Pathol 2013;66(2):79–89.

86. Li CM, Chu WY, Wong DL, et al. Current and future molecular diagnostics in non-small-cell lung cancer. Expert Rev Mol Diagn 2015;15(8):1061–74.

87. Paez JG, Janne PA, Lee JC, et al. EGFR mutations in lung cancer: correlation with clinical response to gefitinib therapy. Science 2004;304(5676):1497–500.

88. Lynch TJ, Bell DW, Sordella R, et al. Activating mutations in the epidermal growth factor receptor underlying responsiveness of non-small-cell lung cancer to gefitinib. N Engl J Med 2004;350(21):2129–39.

89. Shepherd FA, Rodrigues Pereira J, Ciuleanu T, et al. Erlotinib in previously treated non-small-cell lung cancer. N Engl J Med 2005;353(2):123–32.

90. Maione P, Sacco PC, Sgambato A, et al. Overcoming resistance to targeted therapies in NSCLC: current approaches and clinical application. Ther Adv Med Oncol 2015;7(5):263–73.

91. Toyokawa G, Seto T. Anaplastic lymphoma kinase rearrangement in lung cancer: its biological and clinical significance. Respir Investig 2014;52(6):330–8.

92. Gainor JF, Shaw AT. Novel targets in non-small cell lung cancer: ROS1 and RET fusions. Oncologist 2013;18(7):865–75.

93. Yi ES, Chung JH, Kulig K, et al. Detection of anaplastic lymphoma kinase (ALK) gene rearrangement in non-small cell lung cancer and related issues in ALK inhibitor therapy: a literature review. Mol Diagn Ther 2012;16(3):143–50.

94. Rothschild SI. Targeted therapies in non-small cell lung cancer-beyond EGFR and ALK. Cancers (Basel) 2015;7(2):930–49.

95. Masters GA, Temin S, Azzoli CG, et al. Systemic therapy for stage IV non-small-cell lung cancer: American Society of Clinical Oncology clinical practice guideline update. J Clin Oncol 2015;33(30):3488–515.

96. Finocchiaro G, Toschi L, Gianoncelli L, et al. Prognostic and predictive value of MET deregulation in non-small cell lung cancer. Ann Transl Med 2015;3(6):83.

97. Stewart EL, Tan SZ, Liu G, et al. Known and putative mechanisms of resistance to EGFR targeted therapies in NSCLC patients with EGFR mutations—a review. Transl Lung Cancer Res 2015;4(1):67–81.

98. Stella GM, Scabini R, Inghilleri S, et al. EGFR and KRAS mutational profiling in fresh non-small cell lung cancer (NSCLC) cells. J Cancer Res Clin Oncol 2013; 139(8):1327–35.

99. Stinchcombe TE. Novel agents in development for advanced non-small cell lung cancer. Ther Adv Med Oncol 2014;6(5):240–53.

100. Khoo C, Rogers TM, Fellowes A, et al. Molecular methods for somatic mutation testing in lung adenocarcinoma: EGFR and beyond. Transl Lung Cancer Res 2015;4(2):126–41.

101. Tucker T, Marra M, Friedman JM. Massively parallel sequencing: the next big thing in genetic medicine. Am J Hum Genet 2009;85(2):142–54.

102. Popper HH, Ryska A, Timar J, et al. Molecular testing in lung cancer in the era of precision medicine. Transl Lung Cancer Res 2014;3(5):291–300.

103. Deeb KK, Hohman CM, Risch NF, et al. Routine clinical mutation profiling of non-small cell lung cancer using next-generation sequencing. Arch Pathol Lab Med 2015;139(7):913–21.

104. Coco S, Truini A, Vanni I, et al. Next generation sequencing in non-small cell lung cancer: new avenues toward the personalized medicine. Curr Drug Targets 2015;16(1):47–59.

105. Couraud S, Vaca-Paniagua F, Villar S, et al. Noninvasive diagnosis of actionable mutations by deep sequencing of circulating free DNA in lung cancer from never-smokers: a proof-of-concept study from BioCAST/IFCT-1002. Clin Cancer Res 2014;20(17):4613–24.

106. Ilie M, Hofman V, Long E, et al. Current challenges for detection of circulating tumor cells and cell-free circulating nucleic acids, and their characterization in non-small cell lung carcinoma patients. What is the best blood substrate for personalized medicine? Ann Transl Med 2014;2(11):107.

107. Diaz LA Jr, Bardelli A. Liquid biopsies: genotyping circulating tumor DNA. J Clin Oncol 2014;32(6):579–86.

Screening for Lung Cancer

Brendon M. Stiles, MD[a], Bradley Pua, MD[b], Nasser K. Altorki, MD[a],*

KEYWORDS

- Lung cancer • Screening • Thoracic surgeons • Pulmonary nodules

KEY POINTS

- The goal of screening programs is to detect tumors in earlier, curable stages, consequently reducing disease-specific mortality.
- The issue of screening has great relevance to thoracic surgeons, who should play a leading role in the debate over screening and its consequences.
- The burden is on thoracic surgeons to work in a multidisciplinary setting to guide and treat these patients safely and responsibly, with low morbidities and mortalities of potential diagnostic or therapeutic interventions.

Lung cancer is a global health burden and is among the most common and deadliest of all malignancies worldwide. In the United States, lung cancer accounts for more than 25% of all cancer deaths, exceeding deaths from breast, colon, and prostate cancers combined.[1] More than 80% of individuals with lung cancer die of the disease, primarily because a large proportion of patients with lung cancer present with locally advanced or metastatic disease. Intuitively, early detection of resectable and potentially curable disease may reduce the overall death rate from lung cancer. Historically, screening for lung cancer was not recommended by most clinical societies and health care agencies in the United States. However, following the mortality benefit identified in the National Lung Screening Trial (NLST), published in 2011,[2] most US guidelines now recommend screening with low-dose computed tomography (LDCT) in at-risk populations.[3–6] This shift in policy can be expected to significantly increase the number of patients found to have lung cancer, but also those found to have benign lung nodules. Much of the current debate has now turned toward identifying the most appropriate "at-risk" populations for screening, ensuring appropriate management of screen detected nodules, and defining the optimum duration of computed tomography (CT) screening.

The authors have nothing to disclose.
[a] Division of Thoracic Surgery, New York-Presbyterian Hospital, Weill Cornell Medicine, 525 East 68th Street, New York, NY 10065, USA; [b] Department of Radiology, New York-Presbyterian Hospital, Weill Cornell Medicine, 525 East 68th Street, New York, NY 10065, USA
* Corresponding author.
E-mail address: nkaltork@med.cornell.edu

Surg Oncol Clin N Am 25 (2016) 469–479
http://dx.doi.org/10.1016/j.soc.2016.02.002
1055-3207/16/$ – see front matter © 2016 Elsevier Inc. All rights reserved.

HISTORY OF LUNG CANCER SCREENING
Chest Radiograph Screening

The first lung cancer mass screening project was conducted by Brett in London from 1960 to 1964.[7] Although not a randomized trial, 55,034 men were assigned to undergo either chest radiograph (CXR) every 6 months for 3 years (the screened group), or a single CXR at the beginning of the study, followed by a repeat CXR at the end of the 3-year period (the "unscreened" group). At the end of the 3-year period, more lung cancers were detected in the screened group compared with the "unscreened" group (132 vs 96 cases). In addition, resectability was enhanced in the screened group. Despite these findings, lung cancer–specific mortality was not different between the 2 groups.

In the 1970s, the National Cancer Institute funded 3 randomized trials for lung cancer screening using both CXR and sputum cytology at Johns Hopkins, Memorial Sloan-Kettering Cancer Center, and the Mayo Clinic.[8–10] Again, more cancers were found in the screened groups of patients, and resectability rates were significantly higher in the screened group. Nonetheless, again there was no statistically significant difference in the lung cancer–specific mortality between the screened and "unscreened" populations in any of the trials.

Early Computed Tomography Screening Studies

In the 1990s, increased resolution and data-acquisition speeds of modern CT scanners rekindled interest in screening for lung cancer. Initial findings from Henschke and colleagues[11] of the Early Lung Cancer Action Project (ELCAP) showed that in a high-risk population, LDCT was superior to CXR in detection of lung nodules. Notably, 2.7% of those enrolled in the CT screening program had lung cancer, the great majority of which were stage I.[12] A subsequent report by the International-ELCAP (I-ELCAP) group addressed overall curability estimated through 10-year survival rates of patients found to have stage I lung cancer by CT screening.[13] The investigators reported an estimated 88% 10-year survival rate, markedly higher than survival rates predicted by the current staging system or among those presenting as a result of symptoms. They inferred that because CT screening leads to early detection of lung cancer and because those lung cancers found as a result of CT screening are curable, that CT screening leads to a reduction in lung cancer mortality. Several other groups subsequently evaluated CT screening for lung cancer. A review by Black and colleagues[14] published in 2007 identified 12 studies, including 2 randomized and 10 single-arm observational studies. Significant variability existed in the study populations and in the definition of a positive finding in each. The percentage of positive screenings ranged from 5.1% to 51%. From baseline screenings, 1.8% to 18% of positive findings led to a diagnosis of cancer. Most of the tumors were stage I (53%–100%), with a high resectability rate (>78%). Only one of the studies reported 5-year survival: 76% for patients with cancer detected at baseline screening and 65% for patients with cancer detected at annual repeat scanning.[15]

Screening for lung cancer with LDCT was not universally embraced, however. Bach and colleagues[16] reported the findings from CT screening of 3246 high-risk patients from multiple institutions. The investigators reported a 3-fold increase in individuals diagnosed with lung cancer and a 10-fold increase in patients undergoing lung resection (compared with expected cases). They also found no evidence of a decline in the number of patients with advanced stages of disease or of deaths from lung cancer in the screened groups. The investigators concluded that CT screening may not meaningfully reduce the risk of dying from lung cancer and suggested that CT screening is inherently prone to overdiagnosis, thus exposing patients to unnecessary surgery. The study generated controversy given that the follow-up was relatively short (3.9 years) and that at least 1 of the 3 studies did not require the exclusion of symptomatic individuals, possibly undermining the core concept of screening.

Modeling Approaches to Estimate Mortality Benefit

Given the inability of early randomized trials and prospective studies to prove a mortality benefit to screening, others have attempted to address the magnitude of lung cancer mortality reduction using modeling approaches. McMahon and colleagues[17,18] from the Mayo Clinic used 1520 current or former smokers undergoing CT screening to model predicted cases of lung cancer and deaths, which were compared with a simulated unscreened control arm. The model ultimately simulated 500,000 cases per study arm based on 5 annual screening examinations, to generate precise estimates of mortality. At 6 year follow-up, the screening arm had an estimated 37% relative increase in lung cancer detection compared with the simulated control arm and a 28% relative reduction in cumulative lung cancer–specific mortality. Although the model included many assumptions, such as lung cancer incidence rates, adherence to the screening protocol, and treatment by established guidelines, the study made a compelling argument for a mortality benefit from CT screening.

Similarly, Foy and colleagues[18] used a lung cancer mortality model developed within the Cancer Intervention and Surveillance Modeling Network (CISNET) to address the potential for mortality reduction by CT screening for lung cancer. The comparison matched members of a CT screening trial (New York-ELCAP) with age, sex, and tobacco exposure–matched control patients from the CARET (Beta-Carotene and Retinol Efficacy Trial), with well-established lung cancer incidence rates.[19] The simulation was repeated 5000 times to compare expected lung cancer mortality between the 2 groups. With the caveat of the inherent assumptions made for the purposes of modeling, the study suggested a 45.6% relative reduction in lung cancer mortality in the group of patients screened with CT.

More recently, a modeling study was performed by the CISNET on behalf of the US Preventive Services Task Force (USPTF). Models were created using deidentified data from the NLST and the Prostate, Lung, Colorectal, and Ovarian Cancer Screening trial.[20] The investigators judged a strategy of screening patients aged 55 to 80, with at least 30 pack-years, and no more than 15 years since quitting as the optimal scenario balancing benefits and harms. In this scenario, the estimated reduction in lung cancer morality is between 8.6% and 23.5%. All of these studies, albeit models, suggested that LDCT screening protocols, logically followed by earlier treatment of lung cancer, do likely provide a mortality benefit.

The Gold Standard: the National Lung Screening Trial

Between 2002 and 2009, the NLST enrolled 53,456 individuals between the ages of 55 and 74.[2] All had a history of smoking of at least 30 pack-years and were either current smokers or former smokers who had quit within the past 15 years. Most individuals were male (59%) and younger than 65 years (73%). The trial compared low-dose CT screening (26,723) to CXR screening (27,733) using 3 annual screening rounds with 8 years of follow-up. In the CT screening arm, there were 354 deaths from lung cancer, compared with 442 in the CXR group, translating into a 20.3% reduction in lung cancer–related mortality. In addition, there was a 7% reduction in overall mortality in the CT arm of the trial. This absolute mortality reduction was unprecedented in the history of lung cancer screening and was greeted with much enthusiasm by advocates of CT screening. The NLST secondary analyses will continue to provide data over the coming years. In addition, several European randomized trials[21–27] are comparing lung cancer CT screening with no screening. It is expected that pooling the results of these trials and the NLST will further clarify the role for CT screening and better define screening protocols. It should be noted that both the DANTE (Detection and Screening of Early Lung Cancer by Novel Imaging Technology and Molecular Essays)[22] and the DLCST (Danish Lung Cancer Screening Trial)[25] trials failed to show a decrease in lung cancer mortality in the CT-screened patients; however, they were likely underpowered. The largest trial among these, the NELSON (Nederlands-Leuvens Longkanker Screenings Onderzoek) study, has not yet reported end results.

IMPORTANT STATISTICAL CONCEPTS

The efficacy of screening in reducing cancer-specific mortality may be confounded by lead-time, length, and overdiagnosis biases. Although the statistical arguments may be examined from many different vantage points and are sometimes difficult to interpret, they have been well described previously by Strauss.[28] In all screening trials, one must distinguish lead time from lead-time bias. The success of any screening program is dependent on a lead time in diagnosis and treatment; this in and of itself does not present a problem. Bias can arise when short-term survival rates are used to assess the value of screening in populations with and without lead time. Lead-time bias should not affect resectability, or more importantly, curability. In the subpopulations of patients with lung cancer in the older screening trials, there was an increased proportion of 5-year survivors in the screen-detected cases compared with those in the control arms in both the Mayo and the Czech studies.[8,29] The survival curves never converged, suggesting that screening did increase the cure rate of patients with cancer. This mature data imply that lead-time bias does not explain differences in survival between those groups. The I-ELCAP investigators' effort to estimate 10-year survival rates, rather than shorter-term rates, was also an attempt to avoid any possible lead-time bias.[13] The estimated cure rate occurs at the plateau phase of the survival cure, its asymptote, at which point the additional deaths that occur are from competing causes. Ongoing analysis of mature NLST data as well as data from other randomized trials will further help to clarify any potential effect of lead-time bias.

Length bias essentially refers to the tendency of screening to lead to the diagnosis of slower-growing cancers more frequently in the baseline round, because these tumors potentially may have been present for a considerable amount of time before the screening study. For tumors detected only on repeat rounds of screening, this is far less of a concern. A review of the Mayo data, however, demonstrates that survival rates were only slightly better in the prevalence cases when compared with incidence cases (40% vs 33%), those diagnosed at repeat screening.[28] In the I-ELCAP, no distinction was made in survival rates between the prevalence and incidence groups. In the CT screening arm of the NLST trial, 270 (48%) cancers were diagnosed on the incident CT, compared with 379 (62%) following repeat screening (NLST). Survival differences between the 2 groups were not reported, but will be important to evaluate in future reports.

Similar to the length-bias argument, the overdiagnosis hypothesis is based on the idea that screen-detected cancers may be indolent and perhaps even clinically insignificant. The lung cancer detection rates were higher in the screened groups in both the Mayo and the Czech studies. Despite this, mortality for the entire screened cohort in both studies was actually slightly higher. Similarly, in the CT-based study by Bach and colleagues,[16] there was an increased rate of lung cancer detection, 144 cases versus 45 expected cases. Despite this increase in detection, there was no decrease in the expected lung cancer mortality rate. The possibility of overdiagnosis has been used to explain these findings as well as the excellent projected 10-year survival in the I-ELCAP study. Several authorities suggest that many lung cancers detected by screening would not progress rapidly to the point of clinical detection and would therefore be unlikely to account for a meaningful share of deaths among screened individuals.

Perhaps the most challenging aspect of understanding the issue of overdiagnosis is defining the term itself. The phrase is often used synonymously with "pseudo-disease"; this implies that the disease would progress slowly and that the individual would die from competing illnesses long before the cancer becomes clinically significant. This definition may thus encompass patients with lung cancer who die of competing (or accidental) causes to be considered as examples of overdiagnosis regardless of tumor stage. The concept of overdiagnosis was first proposed based on data from the Mayo Lung Project. In that study, there was an excess of early-stage lung cancers in the screened group, yet no difference in mortality. Therefore, it was concluded that those excess predominantly early-stage cancers were overdiagnosed. However, when examined critically, they did not fit the profile of indolent cancers. They were on average 2 cm in diameter, not present on the baseline round, had a median growth rate of 101 days, and were nearly all invasive pathologically.[8] Thus, in the screened arm, lung cancers were far more likely to be identified and cannot be thought of as indolent. The similar disease-specific survival rate between the groups may be explained by the high rate of competing causes of death in the screened group, where the number of cardiovascular deaths was nearly 4 times the rate of lung cancer deaths.

There are several other arguments against overdiagnosis. The first is based on the known epidemiologic evidence. For example, studies reported by Sobue and colleagues[30] and by Flehinger and colleagues[31] have documented mortalities in excess of 80% for untreated screen-detected lung cancers. The high mortality of screen-detected small tumors argues against their presumed indolent or nonfatal nature. In fact, it seems that even the smallest lung cancers are almost always deadly. An analysis by Henschke and colleagues[32] of the SEER (Surveillance, Epidemiology and End Results) database revealed an 87% 8-year fatality rate for untreated 6- to 15-mm primary non–small-cell lung cancer (NSCLC). A more recent review of the California Cancer Center registry by Raz and colleagues[33] examined long-term survival in untreated stage I NSCLC. Five-year overall survival was only 6%, with a median survival of 9 months.

More evidence against overdiagnosis may be found from autopsy studies. McFarlane and colleagues[34] reported that the rate of "surprise" lung cancer at autopsy was less than 1% and that many of these patients had in fact died of those cancers. Another study found a slightly higher (3.3%) rate of lung cancer at autopsy, but deemed none of the cancers to have been clinically insignificant, because lung cancer was thought to be the direct cause of death in more than half of the cases.[35] Further evidence against overdiagnosis may also be found in the I-ELCAP data. Henschke and colleagues[32] reported that for the I-ELCAP screening trial, an expert panel of pulmonary pathologists confirmed that 95% of the patients with stage I cancer had invasive tumors that were morphologically indistinguishable from "garden variety" lung cancers. In addition, a subgroup of the I-ELCAP screen-detected cancers was analyzed for biomarkers using immunohistochemistry and fluorescence in situ hybridization.[36] The molecular alterations were found to be similar to those found in conventionally diagnosed cancers. Of note, all 8 I-ELCAP patients with untreated stage I cancer died within 5 years of screening.

Recently, Patz and colleagues[37] cited overdiagnosis as a potential reason for the mortality benefit in the NLST study. They used modeling estimates to determine that the probability is 18.5% (95% confidence interval [CI], 5.4%–30.6%) that any lung cancer detected by screening with LDCT was an overdiagnosed cancer. The investigators considered that when a bronchioloalveolar (noninvasive in new terminology) lung cancer was detected by LDCT there was a 78.9% (95% CI, 62.2%–93.5%) chance of over-diagnosis. In the NLST, there were 110 bronchioloalveolar cell carcinomas in the CT-screened arm, 95 of which were screen detected. In the CXR arm, there were only 35 bronchioloalveolar cell carcinomas, of which 13 were screen-detected (NLST). Given the lack of longitudinal studies to date, it is impossible to determine whether these were overdiagnosed indolent cancers or whether they would have progressed. The investigators concede that because their model was only based on 3 annual screens and an average of 7 years of follow-up, any estimate of overdiagnosis based on lifetime follow-up scenarios must be treated cautiously. Although the natural history of noninvasive lung carcinomas is not well understood, in general, the balance of both epidemiologic and pathologic evidence does not appear to make lung cancer a good candidate for high rates of overdiagnosis by screening.

CURRENT RECOMMENDATIONS

The American Association for Thoracic Surgery (AATS) established an interdisciplinary task to consider the findings from CT screening trials and provide recommendations applicable to daily clinical practice. Six unanimous recommendations (**Box 1**) were presented and accepted at the AATS 2012 annual meeting.[4] The AATS guidelines recommend screening individuals aged 50 to 54 with a 20-pack history if additional risk factors are present. Recommendations also addressed the need for surveillance with annual LDCT in survivors of lung cancer, the need for patient self-risk assessment, and the need for multidisciplinary evaluation. Importantly, the AATS made no recommendation to stop screening after the 3-year time point used in the NLST, citing lack of scientific evidence for cessation of screening. The AATS also proposed that

---

Box 1
American Association for Thoracic Surgery Guidelines Task Force recommendations regarding low-dose computed tomography screening for lung cancer

1. Annual lung cancer screening with LDCT for smokers and former smokers between 55 and 79 years old with 30-pack-year history of smoking

2. Annual LDCT until the age of 79 in long-term lung cancer survivors to detect second primary lung cancers

3. Annual lung cancer screening with LDCT for smokers and former smokers between 55 and 79 years old with 20-pack-year history of smoking and additional comorbidities that infer increased risk of lung cancer greater than 5% over the following 5 years

4. Multidisciplinary approach to lung cancer screening, evaluation, and treatment

5. Development of a Web-based application for patient self-risk assessment

6. Continue AATS engagement with other specialties to develop and refine further guidelines

Adapted from Jaklitsch M, Jacobson F, Austin J, et al. The American Association for Thoracic Surgery guidelines for lung cancer screening using low-dose computed tomography scans for lung cancer survivors and other high-risk groups. J Thorac Cardiovasc Surg 2012; 144(1):33–8; with permission.

long-term cancer survivors should have an annual LDCT until the age of 79 to screen for second primary lung cancers.

The USPTF recommendations are similar to those of the AATS.[3] They recommend annual screening for individuals aged 55 to 80 with a 30-pack-year smoking history, but suggest discontinuing screening when patients have not smoked for 15 years. The USPTF also addressed implementation of screening programs, smoking cessation counseling, shared decision-making, and standardization of follow-up of abnormal findings. The National Comprehensive Cancer Network (NCCN) has also recommended LDCT screening in selected individuals at risk for lung cancer.[38] High risk is defined as patients aged 55 to 74 years with at least a 30-pack-year smoking history without cessation greater than 15 years prior. They also recommended that persons aged 50 years or older undergo screening when they have at least a 20-pack-year smoking history and one additional risk factor. In addition to the AATS, USPTF, and NCCN, several other groups including the American College of Chest Physicians, the American Society of Clinical Oncology, the American Cancer Society, and the American Thoracic Society have all recommended screening for lung cancer with LDCT scan based on the results of the NLST.

Regardless of the method used to screen patients for lung cancer, controversy over the value and best paradigm of screening will likely continue to exist, much as it does for other cancers, including breast and prostate cancer. In 2009, the USPSTF released new recommendations for breast cancer screening, which were quite different from their 2002 recommendations.[39] The Task Force raised the recommended age to begin screening from 40 years to 50 years and recommended stopping screening at age 74. These recommendations generated significant national controversy. The USPSTF's interpretation of the screening data was subsequently refuted by some investigators, who continued to claim a benefit for screening in the 40- to 84-year age range.[40] Similarly, the value of screening for prostate cancer has also been called into question by the results of 2 disparate landmark studies.[41] The European Randomized Study of Screening for Prostate Cancer reported a statistically significant cancer-specific mortality reduction of 20% favoring prostate-specific antigen-based screening.[42] In contrast, the Prostate, Lung, Colorectal, and Ovarian Cancer Screening Trial showed no mortality reduction.[43] Undoubtedly, different structures of competing clinical trials, heterogenous "unscreened" populations, and evolving technological advances will also continue to make an absolute application of the data for lung cancer screening to clinical practice difficult.

RESECTION OF SCREEN-DETECTED LUNG CANCER

To date, lobectomy remains the standard of care for the management of NSCLC. However, the past decade has witnessed a resurgence of interest in sublobar resection for small, peripheral, early-stage lung cancers as well as for nonsolid nodules that are the radiologic manifestations of adenocarcinoma in situ and minimally invasive carcinoma. These lesions are currently detected with higher frequency owing to the more widespread use of CT scanning and the enhanced resolution of CT scanning devices. Their detection will likely continue to increase once CT screening programs are more widely implemented. The rationale for sublobar resection in such instances is supported by the results of several retrospective case series, mainly from Japan, showing that overall and disease-free survival are comparable to those achieved after lobar resection.[27–30]

Recently, Altorki and colleagues[31] reported the overall and cancer-specific survival for 347 patients with clinical stage IA NSCLCs manifesting as solid nodules in the I-ELCAP screening program. Ten-year survival was 85% for 53 patients treated by sublobar resection and 86% for 294 patients treated by lobectomy. Cox survival analysis showed no significant difference between sublobar resection and lobectomy when adjusted for propensity scores or when using propensity quintiles. For those with cancers 20 mm or less in diameter, the 10-year rates were 88%, and Cox survival analysis showed no significant difference between sublobar resection and lobectomy using either approach. Despite these results, most lung cancers detected in the context of screening continue to be treated by lobar resection, which remains the standard of surgical care worldwide.

Currently, 2 randomized noninferiority trials, JCOG 0802 and CALGB 140503, are testing the hypothesis that lobar and sublobar resections are associated with comparable disease-free survival in patients with solid clinical stage IA NSCLC. The role of sublobar resection in nonsolid nodules is also being evaluated in a Japanese phase II trial (JCOG0804) in which patients with either nonsolid ground-glass nodules or part-solid nodules with a solid component of 25% or less were treated with wide wedge resection. Mature follow-up data from each of these trials on survival and recurrence are awaited.

In the meantime, sublobar resection is slowly emerging as a viable alternative to lobectomy, particularly in patients with nonsolid nodules that may represent indolent cancers, namely preinvasive or minimally invasive adenocarcinoma. The challenge in localizing such lesions intraoperatively may be significant, and the application of sublobar resection in such cases requires careful planning. An important aspect of such planning is the participation of an expert pulmonary pathologist who will be able to confirm on frozen section examination the diagnosis of cancer and the adequacy of the resection margins.

The role of sublobar resection in solid lesions is more controversial and should probably be limited to patients with limited cardiopulmonary reserve until the results of the randomized trials are available. However, when sublobar resection is attempted, the surgeon must ensure the absence of nodal metastases in the mediastinal and major hilar lymph nodes. The presence of nodal metastases should prompt conversion to lobectomy. Particular attention should also be directed to obtaining a satisfactory resection margin that is at least equivalent to the greatest diameter of the tumor and is confirmed to be free of disease on the frozen section examination. Such examinations can be challenging for pathologists, particularly for preinvasive and minimally invasive adenocarcinoma. In the absence of a qualified pathologist, an attempt should be made to obtain a wider margin around the tumor. Most thoracic surgeons emphasize the role of mediastinal nodal dissection or systematic mediastinal nodal sampling in the treatment of clinical stage IA NSCLC that manifests as a solid nodule. The merits of mediastinal nodal dissection in the case of nonsolid nodules are less clear because nodal metastases are rarely found in such instances.

Regardless of the extent of parenchymal resection and nodal dissection, minimally invasive approaches are strongly encouraged. Multiple studies have shown that video-assisted lobectomy and segmentectomy are oncologically equivalent to open thoracotomy approaches and are associated with significantly lower cardiopulmonary morbidity, less need for blood transfusion, and shorter length of hospital stay.[32–34] In addition, data suggest that in the context of screening the use of minimal access surgery would be associated with improved cost-effectiveness.[35]

SUMMARY

Lung cancer continues to be a deadly disease. The goal of screening programs is to detect tumors in earlier, curable stages, consequently reducing disease-specific mortality. The issue of screening has great relevance to thoracic surgeons, who should play a leading role in the debate over screening and its consequences. Screening is especially important because screening protocols may generate a 10-fold increase in the number of patients presenting for surgical resection.[16] The burden is on thoracic surgeons to work in a multidisciplinary setting to guide and treat these patients safely and responsibly, with low morbidities and mortalities of potential diagnostic or therapeutic interventions.

REFERENCES

1. Siegel R, Ma J, Zou Z, et al. Cancer statistics, 2014. CA Cancer J Clin 2014;64(1): 9–29.
2. National Lung Screening Trial Research Team, Aberle DR, Adams AM, et al. Reduced lung-cancer mortality with low-dose computed tomographic screening. N Engl J Med 2011;365(5):395–409.
3. Moyer V. Screening for lung cancer: U.S. preventive services task force recommendation statement. Ann Intern Med 2014;160(5):330–8.
4. Jaklitsch M, Jacobson F, Austin J, et al. The American Association for Thoracic Surgery guidelines for lung cancer screening using low-dose computed tomography scans for lung cancer survivors and other high-risk groups. J Thorac Cardiovasc Surg 2012;144(1):33–8.
5. Wender R, Fontham E, Barrera E, et al. American Cancer Society lung cancer screening guidelines. CA Cancer J Clin 2013;63(2):106–17.
6. Field JK, Aberle DR, Altorki N, et al. The International Association Study Lung Cancer (IASLC) Strategic Screening Advisory Committee (SSAC) response to the USPSTF recommendations. J Thorac Oncol 2014;9(2):141–3.
7. Brett GZ. The value of lung cancer detection by six-monthly chest radiographs. Thorax 1968;4:414–20.
8. Fontana RS, Sanderson DR, Taylor WF, et al. Early lung cancer detection: results of the initial (prevalence) radiologic and cytologic screening in the Mayo Clinic study. Am Rev Respir Dis 1984;130(4):561–5.
9. Melamed MR, Flehinger BJ, Zaman MB, et al. Screening for early lung cancer. Results of the Memorial Sloan-Kettering study in New York. Chest 1984;86(1): 44–53.
10. Tockman M. Survival and mortality from lung cancer in a screened population: the Johns Hopkins study. Chest 1986;89:325s.
11. Henschke CI, McCauley DI, Yankelevitz DF, et al. Early lung cancer action project: overall design and findings from baseline screening. Lancet 1999; 354(9173):99–105.
12. Henschke CI, McCauley DI, Yankelevitz DF, et al. Early lung cancer action project: a summary of the findings on baseline screening. Oncologist 2001;6(2): 147–52.
13. Henschke CI, Yankelevitz DF, Libby DM, et al. Survival of patients with stage I lung cancer detected on CT screening. N Engl J Med 2006;355(17):1763–71.
14. Black C, de Verteuil R, Walker S, et al. Population screening for lung cancer using computed tomography, is there evidence of clinical effectiveness? A systematic review of the literature. Thorax 2007;62(2):131–8.
15. Sobue T, Moriyama N, Kaneko M, et al. Screening for lung cancer with low-dose helical computed tomography: anti-lung cancer association project. J Clin Oncol 2002;20(4):911–20.

16. Bach PB, Jett JR, Pastorino U, et al. Computed tomography screening and lung cancer outcomes. JAMA 2007;297(9):953–61.

17. McMahon PM, Kong CY, Johnson BE, et al. Estimating long-term effectiveness of lung cancer screening in the Mayo CT screening study. Radiology 2008;248(1): 278–87.

18. Foy M, Yip R, Chen X, et al. Modeling the mortality reduction due to computed tomography screening for lung cancer. Cancer 2011;117(12):2703–8.

19. Goodman GE, Thornquist MD, Balmes J, et al. The beta-carotene and retinol efficacy trial: incidence of lung cancer and cardiovascular disease mortality during 6-year follow-up after stopping beta-carotene and retinol supplements. J Natl Cancer Inst 2004;96(23):1743–50.

20. de Koning HJ, Meza R, Plevritis SK, et al. Benefits and harms of computed tomography lung cancer screening strategies: a comparative modeling study for the U.S. preventive services task force. Ann Intern Med 2014;160(5):311–20.

21. Pastorino U, Bellomi M, Landoni C, et al. Early lung-cancer detection with spiral CT and positron emission tomography in heavy smokers: 2-year results. Lancet 2003;362(9384):593–7.

22. Infante M, Lutman FR, Cavuto S, et al. Lung cancer screening with spiral CT: baseline results of the randomized DANTE trial. Lung Cancer 2008;59(3):355–63.

23. Lopes Pegna A, Picozzi G, Falaschi F, et al. Four-year results of low-dose CT screening and nodule management in the ITALUNG trial. J Thorac Oncol 2013; 8(7):866–75.

24. van Klaveren RJ, Oudkerk M, Prokop M, et al. Management of lung nodules detected by volume CT scanning. N Engl J Med 2009;361(23):2221–9.

25. Pedersen JH, Ashraf H, Dirksen A, et al. The Danish randomized lung cancer CT screening trial–overall design and results of the prevalence round. J Thorac Oncol 2009;4(5):608–14.

26. Becker N, Motsch E, Gross ML, et al. Randomized study on early detection of lung cancer with MSCT in Germany: study design and results of the first screening round. J Cancer Res Clin Oncol 2012;138(9):1475–86.

27. Baldwin DR, Duffy SW, Wald NJ, et al. UK lung screen (UKLS) nodule management protocol: modelling of a single screen randomised controlled trial of low-dose CT screening for lung cancer. Thorax 2011;66(4):308–13.

28. Strauss GM. Randomized population trials and screening for lung cancer: breaking the cure barrier. Cancer 2000;89(11 Suppl):2399–421.

29. Kubík A, Polák J. Lung cancer detection. Results of a randomized prospective study in Czechoslovakia. Cancer 1986;57(12):2427–37.

30. Sobue T, Suzuki T, Naruke T. A case-control study for evaluating lung-cancer screening in Japan. Int J Cancer 1992;50(2):230–7.

31. Altorki NK, Yip R, Hanaoka T, et al. Sublobar resection is equivalent to lobectomy for clinical stage 1A lung cancer in solid nodules. J Thorac Cardiovasc Surg 2014;147(2):754–62.

32. Henschke CI, Wisnivesky JP, Yankelevitz DF, et al. Small stage I cancers of the lung: genuineness and curability. Lung Cancer 2003;39(3):327–30.

33. Raz DJ, Zell JA, Ou SH, et al. Natural history of stage I non-small cell lung cancer: implications for early detection. Chest 2007;132(1):193–9.

34. McFarlane MJ, Feinstein AR, Wells CK. Clinical features of lung cancers discovered as a postmortem "surprise". Chest 1986;90(4):520–3.

35. Burton EC, Troxclair DA, Newman WP 3rd. Autopsy diagnoses of malignant neoplasms: how often are clinical diagnoses incorrect? JAMA 1998;280(14):1245–8.

36. Pajares MJ, Zudaire I, Lozano MD, et al. Molecular profiling of computed tomography screen-detected lung nodules shows multiple malignant features. Cancer Epidemiol Biomarkers Prev 2006;15(2):373–80.
37. Patz EF Jr, Campa MJ, Gottlin EB, et al. Panel of serum biomarkers for the diagnosis of lung cancer. J Clin Oncol 2007;25(35):5578–83.
38. NCCN clinical practice guidelines in oncology: lung cancer screening. Version 1. Available at: http://www.respiratory-thessaly.gr/assets/lung_screening%201.2013.pdf2013. Accessed August 7, 2013.
39. U.S. Preventive Services Task Force. Screening for breast cancer: U.S. preventive services task force recommendation statement. Ann Intern Med 2009;151:716–26.
40. Hendrick RE, Helvie MA. United States Preventive Services Task Force screening mammography recommendations: science ignored. AJR Am J Roentgenol 2011;196:W112–6.
41. Eckersberger E, Finkelstein J, Sadri H, et al. Screening for prostate cancer: a review of the ERSPC and PLCO trials. Rev Urol 2009;11(3):127–33.
42. Schröder FH, Hugosson J, Roobol MJ, et al. Screening and prostate-cancer mortality in a randomized European study. N Engl J Med 2009;360(13):1320–8.
43. Andriole GL. Update of the prostate, lung, colorectal, and ovarian cancer screening trial. Recent Results Cancer Res 2014;202:53–7.

Bronchoscopy
Diagnostic and Therapeutic for Non–Small Cell Lung Cancer

 CrossMark

Thomas L. Bauer, MD[a],*, David B. Berkheim, MD[b]

KEYWORDS

- Bronchoscopy • Endobronchial ultrasound • Navigational bronchoscopy
- Autofluorescence • Ablative therapies • Airway stents

KEY POINTS

- Bronchoscopy is a minimally invasive procedure that is versatile, has few complications, and can be both diagnostic and therapeutic.
- With proper training, endobronchial ultrasound (EBUS) and electromagnetic navigational bronchoscopy (ENB) have as good if not better diagnostic results than their more invasive counterparts (mediastinoscopy and transthoracic image-guided biopsy).
- Therapies can be delivered to centrally located airway cancers via the bronchoscope, although, for now, these are palliative in nature.

There is more hope with the bronchoscope.

—Shigeto Ikeda

INTRODUCTION

In today's modern medical market where patients and payers want more for less, bronchoscopy has emerged as a primary tool for the diagnosis and therapy of non–small cell lung cancer (NSCLC). It requires no incisions, often requires minimal sedation, and can be performed in an outpatient setting. Flexible bronchoscopy continues to push the boundaries of diagnosing central lung lesions, peripheral lung lesions, and enlarged or metabolically active mediastinal lymph nodes. It has also become the primary tool in delivering palliative therapeutic treatments to patients with obstructive or bleeding central lung masses.

The authors have nothing to disclose.

[a] Thoracic Surgery, Thoracic Oncology Program, Jersey Shore University Medical Center, Meridian Health, 1945 State Route 33, Ackerman 549, Neptune, NJ 07753, USA; [b] Department of Surgery, Christiana Care Health Systems, 4745 Ogletown Stanton Road, Newark, DE 19718, USA
* Corresponding author. Thoracic Oncology Program, Jersey Shore University Medical Center, Meridian Health, 1945 State Route 33, Ackerman 549, Neptune, NJ 07753.
E-mail address: tbauer@meridianhealth.com

NON–SMALL CELL LUNG CANCER

As one of the deadliest cancers, more people die from bronchogenic cancer than from colon, breast, and prostate cancers combined each year in the United States. The American Cancer Society estimates approximately 221,200 new cases of lung cancer will be diagnosed in 2015. They also estimate approximately 158,040 deaths from lung cancer in 2015.[1] This article focuses on the diagnosis and treatment of NSCLC using the bronchoscope.

NSCLC comprises approximately 85% of all lung cancers[2]; 50% to 60% of lung carcinomas are found in the periphery of the lungs. Up to 20% are found in the central zones, and the rest are in the segmental zones. In 1961, an autopsy study showed the 15% of those who died of lung cancer had carcinoma in situ in a synchronous more central location.[3] This potentially has implications for some of the diagnostic features of newer diagnostic bronchoscopes techniques (discussed later).

GENERAL BRONCHOSCOPY: RIGID AND FLEXIBLE

Dr Gustav Killian of Germany first used bronchoscopy to extract a piece of bone from the proximal airway in 1897. Killian went on many more times to use direct rigid bronchoscopy to remove other various foreign bodies as well as to perform examinations on volunteers to further educate himself on the living anatomy of the airway.[4] He used rigid bronchoscopy, which is a fashioned long metal tube that has a large working channel with an internal lumen size of 6 mm to 8 mm. This working channel allows for direct visualization as well as biopsy and suction access. Rigid bronchoscopes also have a separate lumen to ventilate the patient using jet or standard techniques under general anesthesia. The patient is positioned supine with the head extended. A mouth guard is placed for protection of the patient's front teeth as the scope is advanced through the mouth, past the oropharynx, and under the epiglottis and traverses the vocal cords.

Today, the rigid bronchoscope remains a vital technique in the diagnosis and treatment of NSCLC. Despite this, its use in patients with massive hemoptysis and central airway mass is still valuable. Advantages of rigid bronchoscopy over flexible bronchoscopy are mostly all due to its large working channel. The scope itself can then be used as an airway pushing passed obstructing masses. As such, it is recommended that a rigid bronchoscopy set be in the room whenever flexible bronchoscopy is performed for a central airway or potentially obstructing mass.[5,6]

In 1967, Shigeto Ikeda introduced the first flexible bronchoscope. As its name implies, this instrument is pliable and conforms to the twists and turns of the bronchial tree.[4] This is achievable by having the image brought to the eyepiece via bundled thin glass cables known as fiber optics. This leads to many advantages, not least of which is segmental visualization and biopsy.

The benefits of flexible compared with rigid bronchoscopy are numerous, including but not limited to patient comfort, improved diagnostics, and improved delivery of therapies. General anesthesia is not a requirement. Lack of cervical mobility can easily be navigated with flexible bronchoscopy. Also, ongoing ventilator dependence is a contraindication of rigid bronchoscopy, but a flexible bronchoscope can be advanced through an 8.0 or 8.5 endotracheal tube usually without compromising ventilation.

Instrumentation has been made for the working channel of larger flexible bronchoscopes. Fluid can be flushed through these working ports for bronchoalveolar lavage for Gram stain and cultures as well as for cytology. Brushes, forceps, snares, cautery, freezing, ultrasound probes, and needles have all been made for the purpose of either diagnostics of the airway or therapeutic interventions.

ENDOBRONCHIAL DIAGNOSIS OF NON–SMALL CELL LUNG CANCER
Endobronchial Ultrasound

Treatment of NSCLC hinges on its stage at the time of diagnosis and as such the assessment of nodal disease is of utmost importance. Prior to the advent of endobronchial biopsy, nodal status had been determined by a surgical incision or imaging. Suspicious nodes on imaging necessitate a tissue diagnosis. This had either been done via thoracotomy, video-assisted thoracic surgery, Chamberlain procedure (anterior mediastinoscopy), or mediastinoscopy.

EBUS takes the visualization of standard white light bronchoscopy (WLB) and adds an ultrasound feature at the tip of the scope (**Fig. 1**). Linear EBUS has the ultrasound probe tip of the scope whereas radial miniprobe EBUS is an additional piece placed through the working channel of the scope. A radial miniprobe can reach the smaller diameter bronchioles in the periphery of the lung and identify lesions using its small spinning ultrasound probe. This projects as a circular image. After a certain point, the miniprobe is necessarily advanced blindly through the bronchial tree, looking for the changes in echotexture, which signify a pulmonary mass. Diagnostic yield is enhanced with simultaneous use of fluoroscopy. A retrospective study recently showed there are certain CT findings on preoperative imaging that also increase diagnostic yield. These are lesions greater than 2 cm, lesions in certain segments (1, 3, and 6), and lesions closer to the carina, which all have statistically increased diagnostic yields of 70%, 65% to 71%, and 74%, respectively.[7]

Accurate mediastinal staging remains important. Patients with proved stage IIIa lung cancer are more likely to undergo neoadjuvant therapy prior to their surgical resection. Newer technologies, such as navigational bronchoscopy, have increased the results of radial miniprobe EBUS by guiding the probe to a specific airway. Linear EBUS plays a large role in the staging of NSCLC and has changed the face of mediastinal nodal biopsy within the past 10 years.

Linear EBUS has a probe mounted on the end of a traditional flexible bronchoscope. A balloon around the probe is filled with saline to improve ultrasound conduction. A fine-needle aspiration needle, or more recently a larger-caliber needle that can take core size samples, can be placed in the working channel of the bronchoscope while the balloon is inflated. The needle traverses the bronchial wall at an angle and is seen within

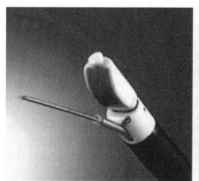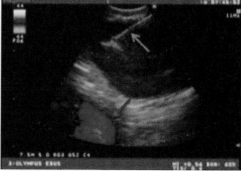

Fig. 1. The image on the left shows an EBUS probe and biopsy needle and the image on the right shows an ultrasound image with biopsy needle (*blue arrow*) within a lymph node well away from the vascular structures (*red arrow*). (*From* Ernst A, Feller-Koopman D, Herth F. Endobronchial ultrasound in the diagnosis and staging of lung cancer and other thoracic tumors. Semin Thorac Cardiovasc Surg 2007;19:203–4; with permission.)

the images produced by the convex EBUS probe. This technique can easily access lymph nodes in the stations 2, 3 posterior, 4, 7, 10, and often 11.[8]

The depth of the biopsy needle can be adjusted, as it is easily seen on the ultrasound image. Vascular structures have an absence of echotexture and are avoided. Duplex features also delineate flow through vessels, making them easily identifiable.[9] In a 2008 study from Lee and colleagues,[10] the number of aspirations taken from each mediastinal sample was shown to contribute to diagnostic yield. The sensitivity of EBUS with 3 aspiration attempts was 95.3% and the specificity was 100%. This was significantly increased compared with 1 or 2 aspiration attempts, with sensitivities of 69.8% and 83.7%, respectively.

A recent study from Toronto compared EBUS–transbronchial needle aspiration (TBNA) and mediastinoscopy in a prospective fashion. All 153 eligible patients received EBUS-TBNA, then mediastinoscopy. Both procedures were comparable in their ability to assess the status of mediastinal nodes. EBUS-TBNA had a sensitivity and specificity of 81% and 100%, respectively, whereas those of mediastinoscopy were 79% and 100%, respectively.[11] Because EBUS biopsy is much less invasive, it is reasonable to perform this procedure instead of the more traditional mediastinoscopy. This is dependent on the experience of the physician and infrastructure of the institution.[12]

Although EBUS is less invasive then surgical staging, imaging could provide improved staging less invasively. Combined and sequential CT and PET scans have both been studied as potential imaging modalities for diagnosing mediastinal involvement of NSCLC. A study from *Chest* in 2008[13] reported the findings of EBUS-TBNA in those with NSCLC and normal mediastinal nodes on CT scan and PET. EBUS-TBNA found positive nodes in 8 patients. Those who were still N0 underwent mediastinoscopy and resection with mediastinal node sampling if warranted. A further 6 patients had mediastinal or hilar lymph nodes positive and 3 patients had N1 disease. All but 1 of the N1 disease patients were identified with EBUS. This study confirms the benefit of adding EBUS-TBNA to imaging and the importance of using mediastinoscopy selectively to accurately determine nodal status without tissue diagnosis.[13]

Electromagnetic Navigational Bronchoscopy

Up to 30% of all lung cancers are in the peripheral one-third of the lungs, placing them in the classification of peripheral pulmonary lesions. Conventional flexible bronchoscopes are typically unable to travel much beyond the segmental bronchial orifice. In the mid-2000s, an advanced bronchoscopic technique was developed that was able to access small peripheral lesions with great accuracy. This system uses computer software that recreates a patient's bronchial tree in 3-D and creates a route from the trachea and ending at the peripheral lesion. The patient is placed on an array mat that creates an electromagnetic field around the patient. This field is able to identify a probe's location placed through working port of a flexible bronchoscope. The combination of all these technologies is termed, *ENB* (**Fig. 2**).

Electromagnetic navigation is used in conjunction with fluoroscopy to confirm accuracy of the biopsy instrumentation. A year after the first human study of ENB,[14] some of the same investigators published an article that put the use of fluoroscopy in conjunction with ENB in question.[15] By eliminating fluoroscopy use, the procedure time is decreased significantly and removes any need for radiation exposure to the patient. They had biopsied 92 peripheral lung lesions using only ENB. The diagnostic yield was 67%. They compared this yields to the 3 previous articles published on ENB, which all used fluoroscopy. These diagnostic yields were 69% to 74%. In this study, diagnostic yield was independent of tumor size. Mean tumor size was 24 mm.[15]

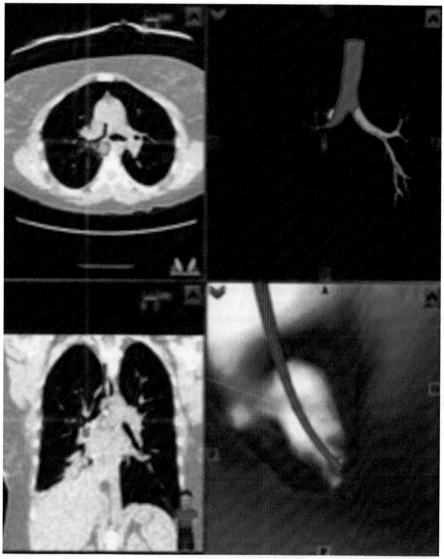

Fig. 2. Example of an ENB screen, (*top left and bottom left*) showing the axial and coronal CT images of a patient and (*top right*) the virtual recreations of the bronchial tree with the route to the lesion marked in purple (*bottom right*). (*From* Backhus L, Puneet B, Bastawrous S, et al. Radiographic evaluation of the patient with lung cancer: surgical implications of imaging. Curr Probl Diagn Radiol 2013;42:89; with permission.)

Other studies show no improvement in diagnostic yield with increasing tumor size. One factor that likely influences diagnostic yield is experience of the user.[16] Although the companies have repeatedly simplified the process, the technology remains heavily user dependent. All the steps from registration to navigation and biopsy are easy to learn but require experience to become proficient.[12]

A meta-analysis from China in 2015 examined the diagnostic yield and safety of ENB; 15 studies were ultimately included in the article. A total of 1106 patients were identified and 1161 lung nodules were biopsied, all using the same ENB system. The diagnostic yields ranged from 59.9% to 94%. Safety was exceptional, with only 2 pneumothoraces in 681 procedures directly attributed to ENB. Seven cases had bleeding associated with them. The investigators also calculated pooled sensitivity and specificity at 82% and 100%, respectively.[17]

Autofluorescence and Narrow Band Imaging Bronchoscopy

Much research has been done to identify cancer in its earlier forms. The idea that cancer follows a stepwise progression from a nonmalignant tissue in the form of dysplasia to a malignant tumor maintains interest in improving today's technologies to help identify cancer at its earliest possible point. It is no different for bronchogenic carcinoma. In a 2001 study, the progression of 416 lesions was followed for 2 years and assessed with the help of fluorescence bronchoscopy. Six of 36 normal epithelial samples became dysplastic. Ten of 27 termed, *severe dysplastic lesions*, persisted or progressed, and 28 of 32 carcinoma in situ sites persisted or progressed. To confound these numbers, some dysplastic lesions also regressed by the end of the follow-up and 1 of the lesions went from metaplasia to invasive cancer.[18]

Additions to the basic features of the flexible bronchoscope have been made since the original visualization via fiber optics. Now, video bronchoscopy is achieved using a white light source and charge-coupled devices, allowing for more detailed visualization of the airway as well as projection of the image onto a monitor for ease of use and education of students. Further advancements have limited the wavelength of both the light source and the filters to help identify mucosal and submucosal lesions.

Autofluorescence bronchoscopy (AFB) was first written about in the early 1990s (**Fig. 3**). Hung and colleagues[19] described spectral analysis of normal bronchial tissue, dysplasia, and carcinoma in situ. First, it was found that tissue with dysplasia or carcinoma in situ had a much lower intensity of autofluorescence when excited with select wavelengths.[19] The subsequent article, published in *Chest*,[20] compared light-induced fluorescence endoscopy (LIFE) with conventional WLB. Because of scatter, reflectance, and absorption, many in situ lesions detected by sputum cytology were unable to be seen with WLB. In this study, WLB detected 35 of the 142 lesions sampled. The addition of LIFE detected 95 of the 142 lesions. The rest of the lesions

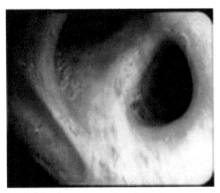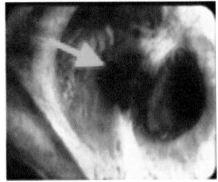

Fig. 3. The image on the right demonstrates AFB detecting an area of carcinoma in situ within the airway (*green arrow*), whereas WLB (white light bronchoscopy) does not detect the lesion (*left*). (*From* Ikeda N, Honda H, Hayashi A, et al. Early detection of bronchial lesions using newly developed videoendoscopy-based autofluorescence bronchoscopy. Lung Cancer 2005;52:24; with permission.)

were detected with random biopsy giving them the label of false negative. The final result of this analysis was that the relative sensitivity of WLB plus LIFE versus WLB alone was 2.71. The relative sensitivity of WLB plus LIFE versus WLB alone for intra-epithelial lesions containing moderate dysplasia or carcinoma in situ was 6.3.[20]

More recently, autofluoresence bronchoscopy plus WLB versus WLB alone was compared in a 2005 study in Europe. This study used had data from 8 different institutions and covered the span of 4 years. This randomized prospective trial reported on a sensitivity of WLB plus AFB of 82.3% and that of WLB alone 57.9%. Specificity of WLB plus AFB was 58.4% and of WLB alone 62.1%.[21] Bronchitis can increase inflammation and dilation of the mucosal and submucosal vasculature and as such can result in false-positive results.

There are 2 improvements to AFB, which have tried to increase the specificity of this diagnostic tool. The first is autofluorescence imaging (AFI), which registers 3 different signals. The signals include autofluorescence when illuminated with a blue light of a wavelength range of 395 nm to 445 nm, reflected light of 550 nm, and lastly reflected light of 610 nm. A Japanese study from 2004 compared this AFI scope to LIFE (the more standard AFB unit) with similarly excellent sensitivities but increased specificity when using AFI. The specificity of AFI was 83.3% whereas LIFE was 36.6%.[22] The investigators were able to achieve this because the AFI unit was able more accurately distinguish between benign and malignant lesions.

Narrow band imaging is another variation of AFB that increases specificity. This bronchoscope uses only 2 narrow wavebands from its light source. It irradiates the surface of the bronchi with blue (390–445 nm) and green (530–550 nm) wavelengths of light. Mucosal capillaries absorb the blue waves whereas the submucosal capillaries absorb the green waves. An experienced practitioner can then distinguish between suspicious and nonsuspicious inflammation. A meta-analysis from 2015, which included a final total of 8 studies, showed pooled sensitivity for NBI was 80% and pooled specificity 84%, whereas if the AFI and NBI were used in combination, the pooled sensitivity and specificity were 86% and 75%, respectively.[23]

ENDOBRONCHIAL THERAPY FOR NON-SMALL CELL LUNG CANCER

Most NSCLCs are advanced stage at presentation.[24] To this end, palliation becomes an important discussion. Not only is bronchoscopy ideal for the diagnosis and staging of NSCLC but also it is an ideal mode of delivering therapies to an often elderly, comorbid population. It requires no incision, has a very short procedure time, can be performed in an outpatient setting, and has few complications. A combination of these interventional bronchoscopic therapies can be advantageous and in a small retrospective trial from 2004 shown to increase 3-year survival from 2.3% to 22% compared with single-modality therapy.[25]

Photodynamic Therapy

Photodynamic therapy has been around for many decades and can be used in the treatment of various cancers, including endobronchial tumors. This therapy takes several days for 1 session and often takes 2 sessions. It relies on 1 of 3 Food and Drug Administration–approved intravenous medications: porfimer sodium (Photofrin), aminolevulinic acid (Levulan Kerastick), and the methyl ester of aminolevulinic acid (methyl–aminolevulinic acid). These medications are given to the patient 1 to 2 days prior to therapy and are selectively retained by malignant cells due to their higher metabolic activity; all cells in the body take up the medication although all do not retain them at the same rates. The medications are engineered to be activated when exposed to a predetermined wavelength of light. A light source is passed through the working channel of a flexible bronchoscope and brought near the tumor. The activated form of the medication is toxic because it creates oxygen radicals. Necrotic tissue is removed from the airway. A few days later, bronchoscopy is carried out to remove the remaining dead, sloughed tissue that remains after therapy and to assess the need for further treatments.[26]

Most side effects of PDT result from all cells in the body absorbing these photosensitive drugs. It is the uniquely high metabolic activity of the cancer cells that allow it to be retained. If a patient is exposed to direct sunlight in those 6 to 7 days of therapy, there may be mild to severe skin irritation. Normal mucosa can be harmed if the light source is not focused onto the area of question. Also, if the area of treatment is near any larger superficial blood vessels, there may be associated bleeding in the area.

Laser Therapy

Laser therapy is yet another way for a skilled practitioner to harness the properties of light to achieve palliation in tumors involving the central airways. The most common form of laser therapy used in the airway is the Nd-YAG lasers because the wavelength of light created by them is able to be transmitted through fiber-optic cables and thus they can be used in conjunction with bronchoscopy. This wavelength (1060 nm) is also the one most biologically active in the airways.[27]

Although the beams can be delivered through a flexible device, laser therapy is often performed under general anesthesia and through the working channel of a rigid bronchoscope. This is for debulking. As discussed previously, the patient populations in whom endobronchial therapy is used in are those who cannot or should not undergo surgery. The laser is used to free the mass from the bronchial wall, thus enabling the tumor to be removed with forceps or with the end of the rigid scope itself (**Fig. 4**).

Cryotherapy

Airway tumors may also be debulked with the application of extreme cold to the tumor itself through cryospray or a cryoprobe. As with laser ablative therapy, it is performed under general anesthesia and with a rigid or flexible bronchoscope. Visualization of the tumor is achieved, and the cryoprobe is placed down the working channel. Nitrous oxide is used to create a goal temperature of -70°C. This process can be done through several freeze-thaw cycles and then necrotic tissue is removed. This can be repeated as needed.

In a prospective trial from the United Kingdom published in *Chest*, investigators showed benefit in outcome measures after endobronchial cryotherapy.[28] More than

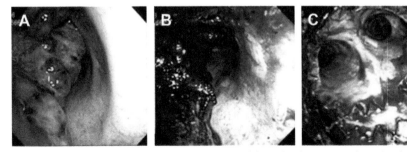

Fig. 4. From left to right, these images capture a (*A*) tracheal tumor undergoing laser ablative therapy (*B*) and stenting (*C*) resulting in a patient airway. (*From* Seaman JC, Musani AI. Endobronchial ablative therapies. Clin Chest Med 2013;34:420; with permission.)

300 patients underwent cryotherapy at a single institution from 1996 to 2000. Approximately half of these patients underwent a conventional 2 sessions whereas the other half were not able to undergo a second session. Cryotherapy has up to a 79% effectiveness of opening an obstructed airway from a malignancy. The ablative therapies discussed previously have similar effectiveness, with photodynamic therapy at 80% and laser therapy at 60% distally to greater than 90% in the trachea.[29]

Stents

Palliation for advanced, symptomatic central lung cancer involves many options. A patient with this pathology may have shortness of breath, hemorrhage, or obstructive processes, including infection, and may benefit from endoluminal stents. These devices have been ubiquitously used in almost all areas of medicine, including cardiovascular specialties as well as gastrointestinal specialties used in the esophagus, biliary tract, and colon. Stents in the airway have been used for many years and may be metal (nitinol) or solid silicone. The metal stents may either be bare or more commonly covered with a thin silastic membrane that prevents tissue ingrowth.

Stents counter the force that a tumor places on the bronchus. Long term, stents can erode through the bronchial wall. These also have increased probability of ingrowth into the tissues they abut and are not easily removed or moved if not fully covered. Silicone stents have less radial force, have a tendency to migrate, and do not have as much ingrowth of the surrounding tissues. As such, they have a tendency to migrate but are much more easily retrievable if necessary. Metal stents should not be left long term in patients with benign diseases.

Hauck and colleagues[30] studied early treatment with bare metal stents placed across either exophytic or external compression of malignant lesions in the late 1990s. In their patient number of 51, they had an initial success rate of postprocedure patency of 91% and a significant improvement in pulmonary function tests. They categorized their complications into early phase and late phase. The most common early-phase complication was mucus retention whereas the most common late-phase complication was tumor ingrowth and what they called "tumor penetration."[30] Other side effects of bare metal stents are cough (which usually resolves within the first couple days), migration, and granulation tissue overgrowth.[31]

SUMMARY

In conclusion, bronchoscopy continues to push the limits of noninvasive procedures. Lesions are identified earlier than ever before. Treatments are deployed to relieve symptoms, and in the future bronchoscopes therapies may be curative. If new bronchoscope techniques and research continue to be used, developed, and funded, lung cancer mortality ultimately may decrease, by helping to diagnose and treat this disease at the earliest opportunity.

REFERENCES

1. American Cancer Society. Internet. Available at: http://www.cancer.org/cancer/lungcancer-non-smallcell/detailedguide/non-small-cell-lung-cancer-key-statistics. Accessed May 1, 2015.

2. Houston K, Henley SJ, White MC, et al. Patterns in lung cancer incidence rates and trends by histologic type in the United States, 2004-2009. Lung Cancer 2014;86:22–8.

3. Auerbach O, Stout AP, Hammond C, et al. Changes in bronchial epithelium in relation to cigarette smoking and in relation to lung cancer. N Engl J Med 1961;265:253–66.
4. Becker H. Bronchoscopy: the past, the present, and the future. Clin Chest Med 2010;31:1–18.
5. Prakash U. Advances in bronchoscopic procedures. Chest 1999;116:1403–8.
6. Simoff M. Endobronchial management of advanced lung cancer. Cancer Control 2001;8:337–43.
7. Guvenc C, Yserbyt J, Testelmans D, et al. Computed tomography characteristics predictive for radial EBUS-miniprobe-guided diagnosis of pulmonary lesions. J Thorac Oncol 2015;10:472–8.
8. Zaric B, Stojsic V, Sarcev T, et al. Advanced bronchoscopic techniques in diagnosis and staging of lung cancer. J Thorac Dis 2013;5:S359–70.
9. Kokkonouzis I, Strimpakos A, Lampaditis I, et al. The role of endobronchial ultrasound in lung cancer diagnosis and staging: a comprehensive review. Clin Lung Cancer 2012;13:408–15.
10. Lee HS, Lee GK, Lee HS, et al. Real-time endobronchial ultrasound-guided transbronchial needle aspiration inmediastinal staging of non-small cell lung cancer: how many aspirations per target lymph node station? Chest 2008;134:368–74.
11. Yasufuku K, Pierre A, Darling G, et al. A Prospective controlled trial of endobronchial ultrasound-guided transbronchial needle aspiration compared with mediastinoscopy for mediastinal lymph node staging of lung cancer. J Thorac Cardiovasc Surg 2011;142:1393–400.
12. Rivera MP, Mehta AC, Wahidi MM. Establishing the diagnosis of lung cancer: diagnosis and management of lung cancer, 3rd ed: American College of Chest Physicians evidence-based clinical practice guidelines. Chest 2013;143:e142S–65S.
13. Herth F, Eberhardt R, Krasnik M, et al. Endobronchial ultrasound-guided transbronchial needle aspiration of lymph nodes in the radiologically and positron emission tomography-normal mediastinum in patients with lung cancer. Chest 2008;133:887–91.
14. Schwarz Y, Greif J, Becker H, et al. Real-time electromagnetic navigation bronchoscopy to peripheral lung lesions using overlaid ct images. Chest 2006;129:988–94.
15. Eberhardt R, Anantham D, Herth F, et al. Electromagnetic navigation diagnostic bronchoscopy in peripheral lung lesions. Chest 2007;131:1800–5.
16. Lamprecht B, Porsch P, Wegleitner B, et al. Electromagnetic Navigation Bronchoscopy (ENB) increasing diagnostic yield. Respir Med 2012;106:710–5.
17. Zhang W, Chen S, Dong X, et al. Meta-analysis of the diagnostic yield and safety of electromagnetic navigation bronchoscopy for lung nodules. J Thorac Dis 2015;7:799–809.
18. Bota S, Auliac J-B, Paris C, et al. Follow-up of Bronchial Precancerous Lesions and Carcinoma in Situ Using Fluorescence Endoscopy. Am J Respir Crit Care Med 2001;164:1688–93.
19. Hung J, Lam S, LeRiche JC, et al. Autoflurescence of normal and malignant bronchial tissue. Lasers Surg Med 1981;11:98–105.
20. Lam S, Kennedy T, Unger M, et al. Localization of bronchial intraepithelial neoplastic lesions by fluorescence bronchoscopy. Chest 1998;113:696–702.
21. HauBinger K, Becker H, Stanzel F, et al. Autofluorescence bronchoscopy with white light bronchoscopy compared with white light bronchoscopy alone for

the detection of precancerous lesions: a European randomized controlled multi-center trial. Thorax 2005;60:496–503.

22. Chiyo M, Shibuya K, Hoshino H, et al. Effective detection of bronchial preinvasive lesions by a new autofluorescence imaging bronchovideoscope system. Lung Cancer 2005;48:307–13.

23. Iftikhar I, Musani A. Narrow-band imaging bronchoscopy in the detection of pre-malignant airway lesions: a meta-analysis of diagnostic test accuracy. Ther Adv Respir Dis 2015;9(5):207–16.

24. Chin CS, Litle V, Yun J, et al. Airway stents. Ann Thorac Surg 2008;85:S792–6.

25. Santos R, Raftopoulos Y, Keenan R, et al. Bronchoscopic palliation of primary lung cancer: single or multimodality therapy. Surg Endosc 2004;18:931–6.

26. Folch E, Mehta AC. Airway interventions in the tracheobronchial tree. Semin Respir Crit Care Med 2008;29:441–52.

27. Dutau H, Breen DP. Endobronchial laser treatment: an essential tool in therapeutic bronchoscopy. Eur Respir Mon 2012;48:149–60.

28. Asimakopoulos G, Beeson J, Evans J, et al. Cryosurgery for malignant endobronchial tumors: analysis of outcome. Chest 2005;127:2007–14.

29. Rand I, Barber P, Goldring J, et al. Summary of the British Thoracic Society Guidelines for advanced diagnostic and therapeutic flexible bronchoscopy in adults. Thorax 2011;66:1014–5.

30. Hauck RW, Lembeck RM, Emslander HP, et al. Implantation of accuflex and strecker stents in malignant bronchial stenoses by flexible bronchoscopy. Chest 1997;112:134–44.

31. Gaafar AH, Shaaban AY, Elhadidi MS. The use of metallic expandable tracheal stents in the management of inoperable malignant tracheal obstruction. Eur Arch Otorhinolaryngol 2012;269:247–53.

Mediastinal Staging in Non–Small Cell Lung Cancer

Ziv Gamliel, MD

KEYWORDS

- Lung cancer staging • Mediastinal lymph nodes • Mediastinoscopy
- Endobronchial ultrasound

KEY POINTS

- In the absence of distant metastases, lung cancer treatment is determined by the results of mediastinal lymph node staging.
- Occult mediastinal lymph node metastases can be missed by radiologic and needle-based staging methods.
- Aggressive staging of mediastinal lymph nodes improves staging accuracy.
- Improved accuracy of mediastinal lymph node staging results in more appropriate lung cancer treatment.
- Improved accuracy of mediastinal lymph node staging can improve stage-specific survival from lung cancer.

IMPORTANCE OF PRETREATMENT STAGING IN THE MANAGEMENT OF NON–SMALL CELL LUNG CANCER

Despite advances in the treatment of non–small cell lung cancer, overall cure rates remain low. Only a relatively small proportion of patients with non–small cell lung cancer is diagnosed at an early stage; most are diagnosed only after there has been spread beyond the lung.[1] The optimal treatment of non–small cell lung cancer is stage specific.[2] Aggressive pretreatment staging efforts often lead to "upstaging," which, in turn, results in improved stage-specific survival.[3]

In staging patients with non–small cell lung cancer, the initial goal is to rule out distant metastatic disease. For practical reasons, this is accomplished primarily via imaging studies. As a rule, these include whole-body PET/computed tomography (CT) as well as brain MRI scans. Typically, suspected sites of distant metastatic disease may be confirmed using image-guided percutaneous needle biopsy techniques.

The author has nothing to disclose.
Thoracic Surgery, Angelos Center for Lung Diseases, MedStar Franklin Square Medical Center, MedStar Harbor Hospital, 9103 Franklin Square Drive, Suite 1800, Baltimore, MD 21237, USA
E-mail address: ziv.gamliel@medstar.net

Surg Oncol Clin N Am 25 (2016) 493–502
http://dx.doi.org/10.1016/j.soc.2016.02.004
surgonc.theclinics.com

After excluding distant metastatic disease in the most feasible way, it is critical to rule out regional spread of tumor to the mediastinum. It has long been known that involvement of mediastinal lymph nodes greatly decreases the likelihood of cure using local treatment modalities (eg, radiotherapy or surgical resection) alone. The presence of mediastinal lymph node metastases makes control of systemic disease the priority, and chemoradiotherapy the mainstay of treatment, relegating surgical resection or stereotactic radiosurgical ablation to "adjuvant" treatment status.

THE TIMING OF MEDIASTINAL LYMPH NODE STAGING

By definition, in non–small cell lung cancer, involvement of mediastinal lymph nodes with metastatic tumor is considered stage III and is associated with a worsened prognosis. In the absence of local symptoms, the focus of treatment for stage III non–small cell lung cancer shifts from local control of the primary tumor to systemic control, that is, the successful eradication of suspected occult micrometastatic disease. The addition of effective locoregional disease control may result in cure.

In patients with mediastinal lymph node involvement, surgical resection of non–small cell lung cancer is unlikely to result in a cure.[4] Preferred treatment involves the use of systemic chemotherapy as well as external beam radiotherapy to the primary tumor and involved mediastinal nodes. Although chemotherapy and radiotherapy are more easily tolerated when used sequentially, concurrent chemoradiotherapy results in improved patient outcomes with a greater likelihood of cure.[5] Survival of patients in whom unexpected mediastinal lymph node involvement is discovered at the time of surgical resection is somewhat improved with the addition of postoperative radiotherapy and chemotherapy.[6]

In selected patients, the addition of adjuvant surgical resection following chemoradiotherapy for stage III non–small cell lung cancer has resulted in improved survival and higher cure rates. The highest rates of cure in mediastinal lymph node–positive stage III non–small cell lung cancer are observed in patients who undergo surgical resection following preoperative concurrent chemoradiotherapy and who are found to have achieved effective eradication of metastatic tumor from their mediastinal lymph nodes[7] and a pathologic complete response of their primary tumor to preoperative chemoradiotherapy.[8]

For medically fit patients with stage III non–small cell lung cancer with mediastinal lymph node involvement, survival is maximized by trimodality therapy that combines chemotherapy, locoregional radiotherapy, and surgical resection.[9] Although postoperative radiotherapy improves the prognosis of patients whose mediastinal lymph node involvement is discovered unexpectedly at the time of surgical resection,[6] the chance of cure is highest in patients who undergo surgical resection following successfully "downstaging" with preoperative/neoadjuvant chemoradiotherapy. Patients who are not successfully "downstaged" by preoperative/neoadjuvant chemoradiotherapy have a poor prognosis that is not improved by surgical resection.[7] In view of the above, the optimal time to identify mediastinal lymph node involvement is before a treatment plan is made rather than intraoperatively or postoperatively. The most recent report of using trimodality in the neoadjuvant setting was by Suntharalingam and colleagues[10] in 2012. Radiation Therapy Oncology Group (RTOG) 0229 was a prospective phase 2 study that looked for the effect of neoadjuvant chemoradiation on mediastinal lymph nodes, survival, and patterns of recurrence. Using weekly carboplatin/paclitaxel and concurrent radiotherapy 61.2 Gy, mediastinal nodal clearance was accomplished in 63% with relatively minimal morbidity and only one postoperative grade 5 toxicity.

CONSEQUENCES OF MISSED MEDIASTINAL LYMPH NODE INVOLVEMENT

Because of understaging, patients with unrecognized mediastinal lymph node involvement are likely to be offered inadequate therapy for their lung cancer. Typically, a failure to identify mediastinal lymph node metastases results in inappropriate surgical resection or stereotactic radiosurgical ablation of the primary lesion without any attention to control of the mediastinal disease and without adequate systemic chemotherapy. Patients who are undertreated for their lung cancer in this fashion are likely to experience either regional or distant "recurrence" of their disease. Because their cancer was treated inadequately in the first place, newly identified sites of disease in these patients actually represent disease progression rather than recurrence. In any case, patients with potentially curable lung cancer who are understaged and undertreated are more likely to die of disease progression.

When mediastinal nodal involvement is unrecognized before a primary lung cancer is removed, there is still an opportunity to discover lymph node metastases by adding mediastinal lymph node dissection at the time of lung resection. This discovery is likely to prompt postoperative adjuvant radiotherapy and systemic chemotherapy. Although such a discovery "after the fact" can lead to more correct staging, the benefits of postoperative radiotherapy are not as great as the benefits of neoadjuvant treatment with preoperative downstaging of disease. The patients who are most likely to benefit from resection of their stage III non–small cell lung cancer are those who have been successfully downstaged preoperatively with neoadjuvant treatment.

The benefit of resecting the primary tumor in the face of mediastinal lymph node involvement with non–small cell lung cancer is relatively low. When mediastinal lymph node involvement persists following neoadjuvant treatment, the prognosis is even worse.[7] There is a significant possibility that offering resection of the primary tumor to patients with active mediastinal lymph node involvement might not be beneficial. Moreover, there is a high probability that such a surgical undertaking is likely to delay the onset of more helpful systemic chemotherapy. In the presence of active mediastinal lymph node metastasis, resection of the primary lung tumor should probably be avoided.

BENEFITS OF PREOPERATIVE DETECTION OF MEDIASTINAL LYMPH NODE INVOLVEMENT

The discovery of mediastinal lymph node metastases in patients with non–small cell lung cancer allows potentially futile lung resection to be avoided and affords an opportunity for needed chemoradiotherapy to be instituted in a timely fashion. Even microscopic involvement of mediastinal lymph nodes with metastatic tumor is associated with a worse prognosis. One of the best predictors of long-term survival following surgical resection for stage IIIA non–small cell lung cancer is complete clearance of mediastinal lymph nodes with neoadjuvant treatment.[7] Patients with the least tumor burden in their mediastinal lymph nodes at the time of diagnosis are most likely to experience successful downstaging with neoadjuvant treatment and are most likely to become suitable candidates for adjuvant surgical resection of their primary lung cancer.

THE IDEAL METHOD FOR PRETREATMENT MEDIASTINAL LYMPH NODE STAGING

In order to achieve the maximum benefit, staging of mediastinal lymph nodes should be undertaken before a treatment plan is made in all patients in whom distant metastatic disease has been excluded. Ideally, mediastinal lymph node staging should be readily and rapidly available, well-tolerated, and relatively noninvasive, safe, inexpensive, and highly reliable. Multiple methods of mediastinal lymph node staging are currently in use. These methods vary in their availability, invasiveness, safety, cost, and reliability. Because the importance of their involvement with metastatic tumor was first recognized, the optimal manner in which to evaluate mediastinal lymph nodes in patients with non–small cell lung cancer has been fiercely debated.

In evaluating the usefulness of any method of mediastinal lymph node staging, it is important to consider sensitivity and specificity. The sensitivity and specificity of any given staging method determine its usefulness in managing a population of patients. With respect to decision-making in an individual patient, however, it is far more relevant to consider the positive predictive value and the negative predictive value. In particular, the higher the negative predictive value of a staging method, the more reliable it is for excluding mediastinal lymph node involvement in a particular patient.

NONINVASIVE METHODS OF MEDIASTINAL LYMPH NODE STAGING

Imaging studies can be used to detect the presence of mediastinal lymphadenopathy. CT has been used alone or in combination with PET. CT scanning is widely available and is relatively inexpensive. CT imaging of mediastinal lymph nodes is best achieved with the addition of intravenous contrast in order to better distinguish vascular structures from lymph nodes and other mediastinal tissue. The use of intravenous contrast may be limited by contrast allergy or impairment of renal function.

The use of CT alone for mediastinal lymph node staging in non–small cell lung cancer relies on abnormal enlargement of the mediastinal lymph nodes as a marker for tumor involvement. Mediastinal lymph node enlargement is not always associated with involvement by metastatic tumor. Conversely, involvement with metastatic tumor is not always associated with mediastinal lymph node enlargement. As a result, the use of CT alone for mediastinal lymph node staging is inaccurate.

Currently, pretreatment staging of non–small cell lung cancer with PET/CT is becoming a standard of care.[11] Although PET/CT can be helpful in identifying unsuspected sites of distant metastatic disease, its usefulness in the pretreatment evaluation of mediastinal lymph nodes is limited. PET/CT imaging measures uptake of fludeoxyglucose (FDG); this uptake is determined by metabolic activity and is only an indirect indicator of tumor. Moreover, a critical mass of active tumor must be present before abnormal FDG uptake can be detected. As a result, PET/CT for detection of mediastinal lymph node involvement with non–small cell lung cancer is fraught with false positive and false negative results.[12]

ENDOSCOPIC NEEDLE BIOPSY OF MEDIASTINAL LYMPH NODES

Since its first introduction, transbronchial needle aspiration (TBNA) biopsy of mediastinal lymph nodes has enjoyed increasing popularity. With refinements in endobronchial ultrasound (EBUS) image guidance technology, this approach has been used with great success for sampling lymph nodes in a variety of paratracheal and peribronchial locations. EBUS-guided TBNA is typically performed under general anesthesia with a laryngeal mask airway. In experienced hands, EBUS can achieve results that are comparable with those of mediastinoscopy.[13]

Using EBUS, in addition to sampling mediastinal (N2) lymph nodes, it is also possible to sample intrapulmonary (N1) lymph nodes, although the importance of obtaining such staging information preoperatively is unclear at this time. Because it is performed through the airways, EBUS is not capable of facilitating biopsy of lymph node stations that are removed from the airway, such as aortopulmonary window (station 5), prevascular (station 6), paraesophageal (station 8), or inferior pulmonary ligament (station 9) nodes.

Using transesophageal endoscopic ultrasonography (EUS) guidance, it is possible to perform needle biopsy of paratracheal (stations 2 and 4), retrotracheal (station 3P), paraesophageal (station 8), and inferior pulmonary ligament (station 9) lymph nodes. In order to maximize the number of lymph node stations that can be sampled, EBUS can be combined with EUS.[14–16]

TRANSCERVICAL MEDIASTINOSCOPY

The use of transcervical mediastinoscopy was first described by Carlens and was subsequently popularized by Pearson and colleagues.[4] Typically, mediastinoscopy is performed under general anesthesia with orotracheal intubation. The procedure is performed through a low transverse 2- to 3-cm incision in the anterior aspect of the neck, just above the suprasternal notch. Unlike needle biopsy methods, mediastinoscopy allows relatively large biopsies to be obtained, yielding more than ample amounts of tissue for culture, flow cytometry, and extensive tumor profiling. The development of video mediastinoscopy has allowed the simultaneous passage of multiple surgical instruments via the mediastinoscope without limiting visualization. Beyond mere lymph node sampling, this approach can be used to perform mediastinal lymphadenectomy.[17]

Transcervical mediastinoscopy allows ready access to paratracheal (stations 2 and 4), pretracheal (stations 1A and 3A), and subcarinal (station 7) lymph nodes. By carrying the dissection more distally beyond the tracheobronchial angles bilaterally, hilar (station 10) lymph nodes can often be biopsied. By extending the dissection more caudally in the subcarinal space, paraesophageal (station 8) lymph nodes are occasionally accessible. Inferior pulmonary ligament (station 9) and prevascular (station 6) lymph nodes are not generally accessible via mediastinoscopy. Although the technique of extended transcervical mediastinoscopy described by Ginsberg and colleagues[18] allows access to the aortopulmonary window (station 5) nodes, the technical challenges and risk of major vascular injury associated with passage of the mediastinoscope between the innominate artery, proximal left common carotid artery, and aortic arch make most surgeons uncomfortable performing this maneuver.

Typically, recuperation from mediastinoscopy requires only 1 to 2 days. The small low anterior cervical scar that results from the procedure is not usually very noticeable. The risk of death from the procedure is less than 0.2%. The risk of major hemorrhage requiring open surgical intervention is less than 0.2%. Injury to the left recurrent laryngeal nerve resulting in hoarseness due to left vocal cord paralysis occurs in less than 2% of cases and is the most common complication associated with mediastinoscopy.

Video-assisted mediastinoscopy allows bimanual dissection of mediastinal lymph nodes and makes it possible to perform true mediastinal lymphadenectomy using the transcervical approach. At least in theory, short of open or thoracoscopic mediastinal lymphadenectomy, mediastinoscopic lymphadenectomy is currently the most definitive way to rule out mediastinal lymph node involvement in accessible lymph node stations.[17,19,20]

THORACOSCOPIC LYMPH NODE SAMPLING AND LYMPH NODE DISSECTION

Many mediastinal lymph node stations are accessible via thoracoscopy. These stations include pretracheal (station 1A and 3A), retrotracheal (station 3P), right paratracheal (stations 2R and 4R), subcarinal (station 7), paraesophageal (station 8), and inferior pulmonary ligament (station 9) nodes. Aortopulmonary window (station 5) and prevascular (station 6) lymph nodes are not reliably accessible via any less invasive method and are best approached thoracoscopically. Because they are located medial to the aortic arch, left paratracheal (stations 2L and 4L) nodes are generally not accessible via thoracoscopy.[21]

Thoracoscopy allows excellent access to all areas of the pleural cavity and is at least as useful as open thoracotomy for performing lymph node sampling or formal lymphadenectomy. Unlike open thoracotomy, recuperation from thoracoscopy is relatively rapid; patients can often be discharged from the hospital within 24 hours of surgery and return to unrestricted physical activity within a week or 2.

Thoracoscopic sampling of mediastinal lymph nodes can be performed as the initial step of any lung resection, whether minimally invasive or open". Before committing to lung resection, mediastinal lymph nodes sampled thoracoscopically can be rapidly evaluated using frozen section histology. The discovery of mediastinal lymph node involvement as a result of thoracoscopic sampling, can prevent futile lung resection from being performed, allowing the patient to commence concurrent chemoradiotherapy with little or no delay. Thereafter, if downstaging is successfully achieved, curative lung resection can be offered with a greater likelihood of success.

ANTERIOR MEDIASTINOTOMY

In 1966, McNeill and Chamberlain[22] popularized a technique of left anterior mediastinotomy via the bed of the resected second left anterior costal cartilage in order to gain access to aortopulmonary window (station 5) and prevascular (station 6) lymph nodes. A completely extrapleural approach is sometimes possible; general anesthesia is usually required. In the absence of any visceral pleural injury and with good hemostasis in effect, a chest tube may be helpful in evacuating introduced air from the pleural cavity but need not necessarily be left in place at the end of the procedure.

Before the widespread use of thoracoscopy, anterior mediastinotomy represented a minimally invasive approach to the aortopulmonary window. Currently, thoracoscopy allows superior visualization and manipulation of the aortopulmonary window (station 5) and prevascular (station 6) nodes as well as the surrounding structures and is generally regarded to be a safer and less morbid approach.

IMAGING VERSUS BIOPSY IN MEDIASTINAL LYMPH NODE STAGING

In evaluating mediastinal lymph nodes for involvement with metastatic tumor, currently available imaging techniques are fraught with false positives and false negatives. On the other hand, the rate of false positive results with lymph node biopsy approaches zero. The key factor in evaluating the reliability of any lymph node biopsy technique is the likelihood of obtaining a false negative result.

There are only 3 ways in which the false negative rate of any mediastinal lymph node biopsy technique can be lowered. The first way is to increase the number of sampled lymph node stations. The second way is to increase the amount of tissue sampled from each lymph node station. The third way is to improve the sensitivity of the method used to analyze the sampled tissue.

TRANSBRONCHIAL/TRANSESOPHAGEAL NEEDLE BIOPSY VERSUS MEDIASTINOSCOPY

There have been multiple published comparisons between bronchoscopic/endoscopic and surgical methods of mediastinal lymph node biopsy. Despite the fact that EBUS-TBNA is commonly performed under general anesthesia, it is regarded as less invasive than mediastinoscopy because it does not require an incision and because the potential for bleeding or recurrent laryngeal nerve injury is quite limited. Despite its lesser degree of invasiveness, it is no less expensive than mediastinoscopy and may cost even more. It does allow routine biopsy of hilar and interlobar (N1) lymph nodes that may not be readily accessible to mediastinoscopy. The utility of pretreatment sampling of N1 lymph nodes has yet to be determined.

When performed together, EBUS-TBNA and EUS-FNA afford access to more mediastinal lymph node stations than mediastinoscopy alone. When these methods provide negative results, the false negative rate can be reduced with the addition of mediastinoscopy.[15,23–25]

RESTAGING OF THE MEDIASTINUM FOLLOWING NEOADJUVANT CHEMORADIOTHERAPY

In the absence of distant metastatic disease, patients with lung cancer involving their mediastinal lymph nodes may benefit from trimodality therapy with surgical resection following neoadjuvant chemoradiotherapy. The risks of mortality and morbidity associated with lung resection following neoadjuvant chemoradiotherapy are increased. Because of posttreatment inflammation and fibrosis, minimally invasive surgical approaches for lung resection are less feasible following chemoradiotherapy. After completion of neoadjuvant chemoradiotherapy lung cancer, patients with persistent mediastinal nodal involvement have a poor prognosis and are unlikely to benefit from resection of their primary tumor. Careful patient selection for surgical resection via mediastinal restaging is especially important in this scenario.

Following neoadjuvant chemoradiotherapy, residual hypermetabolism is often seen in the mediastinal lymph nodes. A decrease in hypermetabolism of at least 50% has been associated with successful downstaging and mediastinal clearance.[26] Nevertheless, PET scans cannot distinguish definitively between posttreatment nodal inflammation and residual viable tumor in the mediastinal lymph nodes.

Because of the difficulty associated with histologic evaluation of irradiated tissue, TBNA biopsies may not provide sufficient tissue to allow definitive restaging of the mediastinal lymph nodes. Similarly, frozen sections can be difficult to interpret. In such circumstances, the most reliable method of mediastinal restaging involves histologic evaluation of paraffin sections of large biopsies of the mediastinal lymph nodes obtained via mediastinoscopy or thoracoscopy.

Repeat mediastinoscopy is typically more difficult and dangerous due to indistinct tissue planes and fibrosis resulting from the initial procedure.[27] The added difficulty of performing a repeat mediastinoscopy also lowers its yield of lymph node biopsies. With increased risk of complications and decreased lymph node yield, the advisability of repeat mediastinoscopy has been called into question. When mediastinal lymph node involvement can be confirmed with EBUS-TBNA in a patient deemed eligible for trimodality therapy, it is prudent to "save" mediastinoscopy for mediastinal restaging following completion of neoadjuvant treatment.

WHO SHOULD UNDERGO INVASIVE MEDIASTINAL LYMPH NODE STAGING?

With the ready availability of PET/CT in developed countries, PET/CT scanning is widely if not universally used as an initial staging method in patients with non–small cell lung cancer. Historically, more invasive staging techniques such as EBUS or mediastinoscopy have been used more selectively. Decision-making about when to perform EBUS and/or mediastinoscopy has been guided by assessments of risk, cost, and anticipated benefit.

Patients with peripheral non–small cell lung cancers measuring less than 2 to 3 cm who do not demonstrate abnormal hypermetabolism in their mediastinal lymph nodes on PET/CT are less likely to have mediastinal lymph node involvement with metastatic disease. As a result, mediastinal lymph node biopsy is often omitted in these patients that are staged "clinically" (ie, by educated guess).[28,29] Nevertheless, "occult" metastatic disease in the mediastinal lymph nodes may be present in up to 10% or more of these patients.[15,30,31]

It might seem prudent to avoid the use of mediastinal lymph node biopsy techniques in low-risk patients with a pretest probability of only 10%, because up to 90% of such procedures would yield negative results. The consequences of missed mediastinal lymph node involvement, however, are potentially great. These consequences include ill-advised or ill-timed lung resection and a failure to cure potentially curable disease.

Although the cost burden of "missed" mediastinal lymph node involvement is difficult to calculate, the cost of adding outpatient mediastinal lymph node biopsy in relation to the overall cost of lung cancer treatment is relatively low. From the perspective of an individual patient, the risk of mediastinal lymph node biopsy is low while the potential benefit is enormous. When it can be performed promptly, safely, and economically, pretreatment mediastinal lymph node biopsy should probably be performed universally.

SUGGESTED APPROACH TO MEDIASTINAL LYMPH NODE STAGING IN LUNG CANCER

The approach to mediastinal lymph node staging varies between institutions and among medical providers but should take into account several key guiding principles. Accurate staging should be accomplished before treatment is initiated. Given present day limitations of imaging techniques, lymph node biopsy is much preferred over mere radiologic staging. Negative mediastinal lymph node staging results are increasingly reliable (ie, the false negative rate decreases) the more lymph node stations are evaluated and the more tissue is obtained from each station.

Distant sites of metastatic disease should be ruled out with a PET/CT scan and, when indicated, an MRI scan of the brain. At this point, suspicious mediastinal nodes should be evaluated with endobronchial or endoscopic ultrasound-guided (EBUS or EUS) needle biopsy. Mediastinal lymph nodes that are negative on PET/CT or negative with EBUS/EUS biopsy can be evaluated more rigorously with mediastinoscopic or thoracoscopic biopsy. In order to complete the staging process, any residual mediastinal lymph node tissue should be removed at the time of surgical resection.

SUMMARY

In the absence of distant metastatic disease, the treatment of lung cancer is often dictated by the presence or absence of mediastinal lymph node involvement. Mediastinal lymph node staging can involve a variety of techniques, either alone or in combination; the consequences of overstaging or understaging can be dire. In general, mediastinal lymph node tissue sampling is preferred over radiologic staging. The reliability of mediastinal lymph node sampling may vary with the technique that is used and with the skill of the operator.[11] Optimal mediastinal lymph node staging should be a multidisciplinary process.[28]

REFERENCES

1. Howlader N, Noone AM, Krapcho M, et al, editors. SEER cancer statistics review, 1975-2012. Bethesda (MD): National Cancer Institute; 2015. Available at: http://seer.cancer.gov/csr/1975_2012/. Accessed April 10, 2016.

2. National Cancer Institute. PDQ® Non-small cell lung cancer treatment. Bethesda (MD): National Cancer Institute; 2015. Available at: http://www.cancer.gov/types/lung/hp/non-small-cell-lung-treatment-pdq.

3. Feinstein AR, Sosin DM, Wells CK. The Will Rogers phenomenon. Stage migration and new diagnostic techniques as a source of misleading statistics for survival in cancer. N Engl J Med 1985;312:1604–8.

4. Pearson FG, DeLarue NC, Ilves R, et al. Significance of positive superior mediastinal nodes identified at mediastinoscopy in patients with resectable cancer of the lung. J Thorac Cardiovasc Surg 1982;83:1–11.

5. Curran WJ Jr, Paulus R, Langer CJ, et al. Sequential vs. concurrent chemoradiation for stage III non-small cell lung cancer: randomized phase III trial RROG 9410. J Natl Cancer Inst 2011;103:1452–60.

6. Robinson CG, Patel AP, Bradley JD, et al. Postoperative radiotherapy for pathologic N2 non-small cell lung cancer treated with adjuvant chemotherapy: a review of the National Cancer Data Base. J Clin Oncol 2015;33:870–6.

7. Albain KS, Rusch VW, Crowley JJ, et al. Concurrent cisplatin/etoposide plus chest radiotherapy followed by surgery for stages IIIA (N2) and IIIB non-small cell lung cancer: mature results of Southwest Oncology Group phase II study 8805. J Clin Oncol 1995;13:1880–92.

8. Rusch VW, Giroux DJ, Kraut MJ, et al. Induction chemoradiation and surgical resection for superior sulcus non-small cell lung carcinomas: long-term results of Southwest Oncology Group Trial 9416 (Intergroup Trial 0160). J Clin Oncol 2007;25:313–8.

9. Albain KS, Swann RS, Rusch VR, et al. Radiotherapy plus chemotherapy with or without surgical resection for stage III non-small cell lung cancer: a phase III randomized controlled trial. Lancet 2009;374:379–86.

10. Suntharalingam M, Paulus R, Edelman MJ, et al. Radiation Therapy Oncology Group Protocol 02-29: a phase II trial of neoadjuvant therapy with concurrent chemotherapy and full-dose radiation therapy followed by surgical resection and consolidative therapy for locally advanced non-small cell carcinoma of the lung. Int J Radiat Oncol Biol Phys 2012;84(2):456–63.

11. Silvestri GA, Gonzalez AV, Jantz MA, et al. Methods for staging non-small cell lung cancer: diagnosis and management of lung cancer, 3rd ed: American College of Chest Physicians evidence-based clinical practice guidelines. Chest 2015;143:e211S–50S.

12. Lee PC, Port JL, Korst RJ, et al. Risk factors for occult mediastinal metastases in clinical stage I non-small cell lung cancer. Ann Thorac Surg 2007;84:177–81.

13. Yasufuku K, Pierre A, Darling G, et al. A prospective controlled trial of endobronchial ultrasound-guided transbronchial needle aspiration compared with mediastinoscopy for mediastinal lymph node staging of lung cancer. J Thorac Cardiovasc Surg 2011;142:1393–400.

14. Dhooria S, Aggarwal AN, Gupta D, et al. Utility and safety of endoscopic ultrasound with bronchoscope-guided fine-needle aspiration in mediastinal lymph node sampling: systematic review and meta-analysis. Respir Care 2015;60:1040–50.

15. Szlubowski A, Zielinski M, Soja J, et al. A combined approach of endobronchial and endoscopic ultrasound-guided needle aspiration in the radiologically normal mediastinum in non-small cell lung cancer staging—a prospective trial. Eur J Cardiothorac Surg 2010;37:1175–9.

16. Vilmann P, Clementsen PF, Colella S, et al. Combined endobronchial and esophageal endosonography for the diagnosis and staging of lung cancer: European Society of Gastrointestinal Endoscopy (ESGE) Guideline, in cooperation with

the European Respiratory Society (ERS) and the European Society of Thoracic Surgeons (ESTS). Endoscopy 2015;47:545–59.

17. Leschber G, Holinka G, Linder A. Video-assisted mediastinoscopic lymphadenectomy (VAMLA)—a method for systematic mediastinal lymph node dissection. Eur J Cardiothorac Surg 2003;24:192–5.

18. Ginsberg RJ, Rice TW, Goldberg M, et al. Extended cervical mediastinoscopy: a single staging procedure for bronchogenic carcinoma of the left upper lobe. J Thorac Cardiovasc Surg 1987;94:673–8.

19. Shrager JB. Mediastinoscopy: still the gold standard. Ann Thorac Surg 2010;89: S2084–9.

20. Zielinski M, Szlubowski A, Kolodziej M, et al. Comparison of endobronchial ultrasound and/or endoesophageal ultrasound with transcervical extended mediastinal lymphadenectomy for staging and restaging of non-small cell lung cancer. J Thorac Oncol 2013;8:630–6.

21. Kim HJ, Kim YH, Choi SH, et al. Video-assisted mediastinoscopic lymphadenectomy combined with minimally invasive pulmonary resection for left-sided lung cancer: feasibility and clinical impacts on surgical outcomes†. Eur J Cardiothorac Surg 2016;49(1):308–13.

22. McNeill TM, Chamberlain JM. Diagnostic anterior mediastinotomy. Ann Thorac Surg 1966;2:532–9.

23. Annema JT, vanMeerbeeck JP, Rintoul RC, et al. Mediastinoscopy vs endosonography for mediastinal nodal staging of lung cancer: a randomized trial. JAMA 2010;304:2245–52.

24. Ge X, Guan W, Han F, et al. Comparison of endobronchial ultrasound-guided fine needle aspiration and video-assisted mediastinoscopy for mediastinal staging of lung cancer. Lung 2015;193(5):757–66.

25. Sharples LD, Jackson C, Wheaton E, et al. Clinical effectiveness and cost-effectiveness of endobronchial and endoscopic ultrasound relative to surgical staging in potentially resectable lung cancer: results from the ASTER randomised controlled trial. Health Technol Assess 2012;16:1–75.

26. Cerfolio RJ, Bryant AS, Ojha B. Restaging patients with N2 (stage IIIa) non-small cell lung cancer after neoadjuvant chemoradiotherapy: a prospective study. J Thorac Cardiovasc Surg 2006;131:1229–35.

27. Call S, Rami-Porta R, Obiols C, et al. Repeat mediastinoscopy in all its indications: experience with 96 patients and 101 procedures. Eur J Cardiothorac Surg 2011; 39:1022–7.

28. DeLeyn P, Dooms C, Kuzdzal J, et al. Preoperative mediastinal lymph node staging for non-small cell lung cancer: 2014 update of the 2007 ESTS guidelines. Transl Lung Cancer Res 2014;3:225–33.

29. Fernandez FG, Kozower BD, Crabtree TD, et al. Utility of mediastinoscopy in clinical stage I lung cancers at risk for occult mediastinal nodal metastases. J Thorac Cardiovasc Surg 2015;149:35–41.

30. Gomez-Caro A, Boada M, Cabanas M, et al. False-negative rate after positron emission tomography/computer tomography scan for mediastinal staging in cI stage non-small cell lung cancer. Eur J Cardiothorac Surg 2012;42:93–100.

31. Wang J, Welch K, Wang L, et al. Negative predictive value of positron emission tomography and computed tomography for stage T1-2N0 non-small cell lung cancer: a meta-analysis. Clin Lung Cancer 2012;13:81–9.

Thoracoscopic Lobectomy for Non–small Cell Lung Cancer

Matthew A. Gaudet, MD[a], Thomas A. D'Amico, MD[b],*

KEYWORDS

- Non–small cell lung cancer • VATS • Thoracoscopy • Lobectomy • Segmentectomy

KEY POINTS

- Video-assisted thoracoscopic lobectomy has developed into a safe and effective treatment for lung cancer and is superior to lobectomy via thoracotomy in many regards.
- Development and further refinement of its technique has allowed thoracic surgeons to perform a wide variety of complex procedures in a minimally invasive fashion.
- With future improvement in optics, energy devices, and anesthesia management, the thoracoscopic technique will continue to serve as the pillar for development of thoracic surgical interventions.

INTRODUCTION

Pulmonary resection as treatment for lung cancer has been performed for more than 100 years. The first lobectomy for lung cancer was described in 1912, but pneumonectomy remained the gold standard for many years thereafter. In the 1960s, lobectomy became widely accepted as an oncologically sufficient operation. As technology advanced, thoracic surgeons took on the challenge of performing complete oncologic resections for lung cancer with minimally invasive video-assisted thoracoscopic surgery (VATS) in the early 1990s.[1] The VATS approach to pulmonary resection has continued to evolve significantly over the last 25 years. In addition to pulmonary resection, thoracic surgeons are using thoracoscopy to perform complex operations on the airway, chest wall, mediastinum, esophagus, and even the certain cardiac procedures. Although there are no multicenter, prospective, randomized, controlled trials comparing pulmonary resection for lung cancer via thoracotomy

Dr T.A. D'Amico is a consultant for Scanlan Instruments. Dr M.A. Gaudet has nothing to disclose.

[a] Department of Cardiothoracic Surgery, Ochsner Medical Center, 1514 Jefferson Highway, New Orleans, LA 70121, USA; [b] Section of General Thoracic Surgery, Duke University Medical Center, DUMC Box 3496, Duke South, White Zone, Room 3589, Durham, NC 27710, USA
* Corresponding author.
E-mail address: thomas.damico@duke.edu

and VATS, the minimally invasive approach has produced excellent outcomes and gained widespread acceptance.

Video-assisted Thoracoscopic Surgery Lobectomy as an Oncologic Procedure

Any operation intended to treat cancer should be undertaken with acceptable risk to the patient while also not compromising complete resection and staging. Since the introduction of the minimally invasive approach, many authors have evaluated VATS lobectomy for its oncologic efficacy, safety, reproducibility, and outcomes when compared with more conventional open techniques. In 1993, Walker and colleagues[2] reported 158 cases of VATS lobectomy with 11% conversion rate, 1.8% mortality, and 3-year survival comparable to lobectomy with thoracotomy. As time went on and experience with the technique grew, more surgeons began to investigate all aspects VATS lung resection. Five years later, McKenna and colleagues[3] reported the results of 298 patients who underwent VATS lobectomy, with a 6% conversion rate and 0.3% mortality. Port site tumor recurrence was reported in 1 case (0.3%). McKenna and colleagues[4] followed this up with a review of 1100 patients who underwent VATS lobectomy and reported a 2.5% conversion rate, 0.8% mortality, 0.57% local recurrence, with a mean duration of hospital stay of 4.78 days. Onaitis and colleagues[5] reported 500 VATS lobectomy cases with a 1.6% conversion rate, a 1% 30-day mortality, and no operative mortality. The 2-year survival for stages 1 and 2 non–small cell lung cancer was 85% and 77%, respectively. More recently, Berry and colleagues[6] performed a retrospective review of nearly 1100 patients (610 VATS, 477 thoracotomy) undergoing pulmonary resection for lung cancer and showed similar 5-year survival between the 2 approaches. This was strengthened by a propensity-matched cohort of 560 patients within this group showing no significant difference between thoracotomy and VATS.

Proponents of the open approach to pulmonary resection for non–small cell lung cancer argue that the VATS approach limits the surgeon's ability to adequately perform complete and accurate staging of the mediastinum, a key component of lung cancer staging and an important element of a sound oncologic operation. Mediastinal lymph node dissection during VATS lobectomy has shown to be equal to open lobectomy by D'Amico and colleagues.[7] In this National Comprehensive Cancer Network's database review, close to 400 patients undergoing VATS and open lobectomy were reviewed and there was no difference in the number of N2 stations and mean lymph nodes harvested. In 2 large metaanalyses, VATS lobectomy has been shown to be safe with a conversion rate of 1% to 2% and oncologic outcomes equal to open lobectomy.[8,9]

Many surgeons who had initially trained solely in open pulmonary resection have taken these data and adapted their practices. Current thoracic surgery residents are gaining extensive experience with a wide variety of thoracoscopic procedures throughout their general and thoracic surgery training. Combined, these have led to increase in the number of lobectomies performed via a VATS approach across the world. In a recent review of the Society of Thoracic Surgeons General Thoracic Surgery Database, 45% of lobectomies were performed with VATS techniques.[10]

Advantages of Video-assisted Thoracoscopic Surgery Lobectomy

In a propensity-matched analysis of a single-institution prospective database, Villamizar and colleagues[11] evaluated 1079 patients undergoing VATS and open lobectomy over a 10-year period. Compared with open lobectomy, VATS lobectomy patients were shown to have fewer major complications, including atrial fibrillation, atelectasis, prolonged air leak, pneumonia, and renal failure. Duration of chest tube and length of hospitalization were shorter in the VATS lobectomy group. Similar findings were reported by Paul and colleagues[12] in a review of more than 6000 patients undergoing lobectomy for non–small cell lung cancer from the Society of Thoracic Surgeons Database. In an even larger review of data from the Society of Thoracic Surgeons database, Boffa and colleagues[13] confirmed that patients with stage I non–small cell lung cancer undergoing resection fared better. In this study, patients who underwent thoracotomy experienced significantly more pulmonary complications (21% vs 18%), atrial arrhythmias (13% vs 10%), and were more likely to undergo transfusion (6% vs 4%) than those who were treated with VATS resection, although the mortality was similar. Even when compared with a total muscle-sparing thoracotomy, 1 surgeon found that duration of stay was less for patient who underwent VATS procedures.[14]

VATS lobectomy has also been shown to facilitate delivery of adjuvant treatment, an important component of treatment for patients with advanced stage non–small cell lung cancer. Peterson and colleagues[15] reported a higher percentage of patients receiving 75% or more of their planned adjuvant regimen without delayed or reduced doses after undergoing VATS lobectomy compared with patients who had open lobectomy (61% vs 40%; $P = .03$).

The cost of VATS lobectomy has been reviewed in a study of close to 4000 lung resections[16] and found to be less compared with open lobectomy ($20,316 vs $21,016; $P = .027$). This study also found the risk of adverse events was significantly lower in the VATS group (odds ratio, 1.22; $P = .019$). Recently, Farjah and colleagues[17] even showed that 90-day costs are lower with VATS lobectomy when compared with open technique, explained by decrease in incidence of prolonged duration of stay (>14 days) and less health care use after discharge.

There is also growing evidence to suggest that patient's immune function is better preserved after VATS compared with thoracotomy, as documented by the release of proinflammatory and antiinflammatory cytokines, immunomodulatory cytokines, circulating T cells (CD4), and natural killer cells, as well as lymphocyte function.[18]

Video-assisted Thoracoscopic Surgery Lobectomy: Impact on Other Pulmonary Resections

As the technique has evolved and experience and comfort with VATS lobectomy has grown, thoracic surgeons have used it in various subsets of patients with lung cancer who in the past may not have been considered candidates for a curative resection or would have required a thoracotomy. In patients with poor pulmonary function, advanced age and small peripheral tumors who cannot tolerate a lobectomy or a thoracotomy, VATS sublobar resection (segmentectomy or wedge) can be an attractive option. The lower risk profile of thoracoscopy has encouraged surgeons to investigate its safety in patients who are at higher risk owing to preexisting conditions, including chronic obstructive pulmonary disease. Linden and colleagues[19] performed VATS wedge resection in patients with a mean forced expiratory volume in 1 second of 26% and reported a 1% mortality rate. To decrease the risk of local recurrence after VATS wedge resection, Santos and coworkers[20] reported the use of brachytherapy mesh placement over the stapled lung margin, which led to reduction of local recurrence from 18% to 2%. In patients with forced expiratory volume in 1 second of less than 60%, Ceppa and coauthors[10] reported a much lower incidence of pulmonary complications ($P = .023$) in patients undergoing VATS lobectomy versus lobectomy with thoracotomy.

Technical and oncologic principles of VATS lobectomy, namely individual ligation of the supplying artery, vein, and bronchus, lymph node dissection, and resection of lung parenchyma with surgical staplers have also been applied to performing minimally invasive anatomic segmentectomy. Schuchert and colleagues[21] reported on 225 cases of anatomic segmentectomy performed by VATS or thoracotomy. Length of stay (5 vs 7 days; $P<.001$) and pulmonary complications (15.4% vs 29.8%; $P = .012$) were improved significantly in patients undergoing VATS segmentectomy. Similar outcomes have been reported by multiple other authors with acceptable survival and local recurrence rates.

Berry and colleagues[22] reported on a hybrid technique of VATS lobectomy with en bloc chest wall resection without rib spreading or scapula retraction. In this series, the technique of VATS lobectomy was used to achieve lung resection, which was followed by a small counterincision to remove the involved ribs en bloc. They reported a shorter length of stay ($P = .03$) in 12 patients with this hybrid approach compared with 93 patients who had a thoracotomy.

Further advanced VATS techniques such as bronchoplasty and sleeve resections have also been reported over the last 5 years (**Fig. 1**). Agasthian[23] reported a case series of 21 patients, 9 of whom had simple bronchoplasty; 8 patients had sleeve lobectomy and 4 patients had extended bronchial resection. All patients underwent hand-sewn closure of the bronchus with interrupted sutures. One patient developed bronchopleural fistula. There was no operative mortality and no local recurrence was reported at 6 months. Yu and colleagues[24] reported on 9 cases from China undergoing VATS lobectomy and sleeve resection without any major intraoperative or postoperative complications.

Video-assisted Thoracoscopic Surgery Lobectomy: Development of Uniportal Video-assisted Thoracoscopic Surgery

Over the years, VATS lobectomy has evolved and various modifications with 2 to 4 incisions have been reported by various leading surgeons across the world. Similar to single incision laparoscopic surgery, thoracic surgeons have evolved and VATS lobectomy has been modified into a single incision access with no rib spreading or multiple ports within the same intercostal space (**Fig. 2**). Wedge resections to complex pulmonary resections have been reported. Over a 10-year period, Rocco and colleagues[25] performed more than 600 uniportal VATS cases. The majority of these cases were for pleural disorders and wedge resections for pulmonary nodules. The authors reported excellent outcomes without any major intraoperative complications. Gonzalez-Rivas and associates[26] reported their first 100 cases over a 2-year period

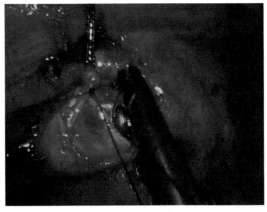

Fig. 1. Bronchoplastic closure after thoracoscopic lobectomy.

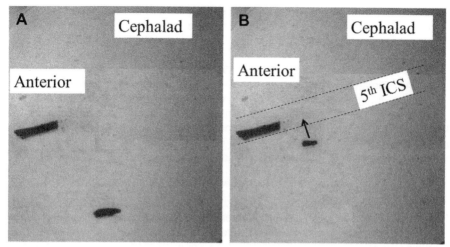

Fig. 2. Traditional 2-port (*A*) and modified Uniportal (*B*) approaches. ICS, intercostal space.

with impressive results. The majority (96%) of lobectomies were accomplished with the uniportal technique, with no operative mortality. Mean chest tube duration and length of stay were 2 and 3 days, respectively. An average of 14.5 lymph nodes were harvested per resection with 154 minutes of mean operative time. Tam and colleagues[27] reported similar results in 38 uniportal VATS lobectomy. Six patients required thoracotomy. In all, 97% of patients did not require intravenous analgesia and mean time to return to full normal activities was 7 days. Gonzalez-Rivas and colleagues[28] have also reported uniportal right pneumonectomy without any major complications. McElnay and colleagues[29] showed no difference in median morphine use or visual analog pain score in the first 24 hours postoperatively, or in patient-controlled analgesia duration, chest drain duration, or overall length of stay in 15 uniportal VATS lobectomies compared with the standard multiport technique.

Video-assisted Thoracoscopic Surgery Lobectomy: Development of Robotic Assisted Video-assisted Thoracoscopic Surgery

Advancement in robotic technology has generated interest among thoracic surgeons to its suitability for VATS pulmonary resections and other thoracic operations. It has been proposed that 3-dimensional optics and the articulation provided by robotic instruments may allow for increased use of a minimally invasive approach for pulmonary resection. The learning curve for robotic prostatectomy has been shown to be the same among laparoscopic trained fellows and experienced open surgeons who are not familiar with minimally invasive skills.[30] This has lead thoracic surgeons to wonder if this experience can be replicated in thoracic surgery. Can surgeons not trained in VATS lobectomy perform robot-assisted VATS resection? More recently, the dual console systems, infrared technology for better anatomic visualization and tissue perfusion as well as improved simulation and training have made surgeons experienced in VATS lobectomy techniques interested in including robotics in their practice. Louie and colleagues[31,32] compared directly robotic and thoracoscopic pulmonary resection in a case-control analysis of anatomic robotic and VATS lung resections: 46 robotic resections (40 lobectomies, 5 segmentectomies, 1 conversion to VATS included in this group for intention-to-treat analysis) were compared with 34 VATS resections (27 lobectomies, 7 segmentectomies). Length of stay, major and minor postoperative morbidity, and operative times were comparable. In a multiinstitutional retrospective cohort study of 325 patients who underwent robotic lobectomy,[30] median chest tube duration and length of stay was 3 and 5 days, respectively. Major perioperative complications were seen in 3.7% of patients and surgical mortality was 0.3%. The estimated 5-year survival was 80%. Implementation of robotic surgery programs carry a high capital cost and require expensive maintenance protocols. In a recent study, Nasir and colleagues[33] evaluated 862 robotic lung resections. The 30-day mortality was 0.25% and major morbidity was seen in 9.6% of patients. The authors estimated a profit of $4750 per patient after factoring in the operative and hospital cost. Median length of stay in this study was 2 days.

Video-assisted Thoracoscopic Surgery Lobectomy: Development of Awake Thoracoscopy

Traditionally, intubation with a double-lumen tube or use of an endobronchial blocker and single lung ventilation has been considered mandatory for thoracoscopic surgery to obtain optimal visualization. This is tolerated well in most cases, but adverse effects of general anesthesia and airway trauma from double-lumen tube placement are inevitable. Many thoracic surgery patients have preexisting comorbid conditions and cardiopulmonary compromise, which makes general anesthesia much more precarious. These issues have led some thoracic surgeons to explore the concepts of awake or nonintubated thoracoscopy. Pleuroscopy with drainage of effusion and pleural biopsy with local anesthesia has been performed routinely with flexible scopes in an outpatient setting for many years, mostly by pulmonologists. Anesthesia for a more complex thoracoscopic intervention, termed 'awake VATS' includes a regional block with or without conscious sedation. This consists of one of the following: local anesthesia, intercostal nerve blocks, paravertebral blocks, and thoracic epidural anesthesia. In this setup, open pneumothorax after trocar insertion leads to gradual collapse of the nondependent lung and leads to spontaneous 1-lung ventilation.[34]

In a small, randomized trial performed by Pompeo and colleagues,[35] 43 patients with spontaneous pneumothorax underwent VATS bullectomy and pleurodesis under a thoracic epidural anesthesia. Their results showed safety and efficacy of this technique of VATS along with shorter hospital stay and reduced cost. The same group has also reported 19 cases of empyema treated with awake VATS decortication.[36] Three patients developed mild hypercapnia that resolved with time and 4 patients required general anesthesia because thick pleural peel required a nonemergent thoracotomy. Chen and colleagues[37] reported their single institution experience of doing awake VATS in 285 cases. Of these, 137 were VATS lobectomy, 132 were VATS wedge resection, and 16 were VATS segmentectomy. Conversion to general anesthesia was required in 4.9% of cases and 1 patient required thoracotomy for bleeding. There was no operative mortality. Anesthesia consisted of thoracic epidural, sedation and temporary intrathoracic vagal blockade for inhibition of cough reflex.

THE DUKE APPROACH

Single-lung ventilation is required and may be achieved with a dual lumen endotracheal tube or a bronchial blocker. The patient is placed in the lateral decubitus position. Most thoracoscopic lobectomies may be performed via 2 or three incisions, and the overwhelming majority in our experience has been performed with only 2.

In general, the port positions are the same whether an upper, lower, or middle lobectomy is performed. The first port, placed in the seventh or eighth intercostal space in the posterior axillary line, is used predominantly for camera placement and, ultimately, chest tube placement. The second port is placed in the fifth intercostal space anteriorly, where the intercostal space is the widest (**Fig. 3**).

Instrumentation is critically important when performing thoracoscopic surgery, including the use a 30° videoscope and long, curved instruments to allow for ease of retraction and dissection. High-definition video equipment improves visualization for difficult dissections. Linear staplers are used to control and divide lung parenchyma, vessels, and bronchus.

Most of the hilar dissection may be performed bluntly, with either a dissecting instrument (**Figs. 4** and **5**) or a thoracoscopic suction device, which also keeps the field dry during dissection, although some surgeons prefer sharp dissection or dissection with an energy device. In most cases, the fissure is completed at the conclusion of the dissection with the stapling device and the specimen is removed using a protective bag. Mediastinal lymphadenectomy is subsequently performed, although this may be done before hilar dissection at the surgeon's discretion.

In addition to the dissection strategy, which varies according to the which lobe is being resected, the surgeon should have a planned strategy for conversion if bleeding is encountered or if there is failure to progress with the dissection thoracoscopically. Most of the bleeding encountered can be controlled with direct pressure using a sponge stick, and that conversion need not be performed emergently.

Right Upper Lobectomy

Once the right chest has been entered, the lung is retracted medially and dissection along the posterior pleura is carried at the level of the bronchial bifurcation, which facilitates bronchial dissection later from the anterior approach. In some patients, bronchial division can be performed at this point. The lung is then reflected posterior and dissection is performed to identify the bifurcation of the upper and middle lobe veins. Once the upper lobe vein has been clearly identified, it is circumferentially dissected free and divided with the linear stapler. This reveals the underlying pulmonary artery. In a similar fashion, the pulmonary arteries to the upper lobe are mobilized and divided, beginning with the truncus anterior. The last structure to be dissected is usually the bronchus; however, occasionally the bronchus is divided before dissection of the posterior ascending artery. After dividing the bronchus, the fissures are developed and divided using stapling devices and the specimen is extracted from the chest in a protective bag.

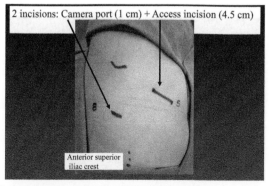

Fig. 3. Location of port placement for traditional approach.

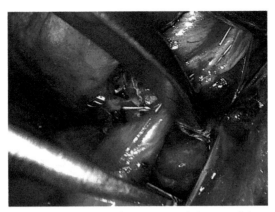

Fig. 4. Isolation of truncal artery during thoracoscopic left upper lobectomy.

Left Upper Lobectomy

Thoracoscopic left upper lobectomy is performed in a similar fashion to that on the right. Posterior dissection is undertaken first to divide the pleural reflection and to identify the posterior artery; as with the right upper lobe, this posterior dissection greatly facilitates the completion from the anterior approach. With the lung retracted posteriorly, dissection is used to identify both pulmonary veins (to ascertain that a common pulmonary vein is not present). The superior pulmonary vein is then encircled and divided, revealing the underlying pulmonary artery and upper lobe bronchus. Dissection of the lymph nodes between the cephalad aspect of the bronchus and the arterial trunk (to the anterior and apical segments) will facilitate the arterial dissection. The branches of the anterior trunk can now be individually exposed and divided, followed by division of the posterior and lingular branches. Bronchial dissection and division is now easily accomplished, and finally, the major fissure is divided with the stapling device.

Left and Right Lower Lobectomy

There are 2 basic strategies for lower lobectomy, both of which begin with division of the inferior pulmonary ligament, followed by dissection and division of the inferior pulmonary vein. The preferred method does not involve dissection within the fissure (which is stapled last, as with upper lobectomy). After dividing the vein, attention is

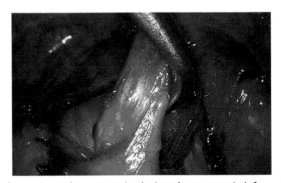

Fig. 5. Isolation of superior pulmonary vein during thoracoscopic left upper lobectomy.

directed to the bronchus by retracting the lobe cranially, a perspective not obtained via thoracotomy. A plane is created between the bronchus and the artery by dissecting close to the bronchus, which is then divided. For right lower lobectomy, this dissection is begun at the bifurcation with the middle lobe bronchus, which must be preserved. The arterial trunk is then encircled and divided, although it is sometimes easier to divide the branches to the superior and basilar segments individually. Ultimately, the fissure is divided and the specimen removed.

SUMMARY

Over the last 20 years, VATS lobectomy has developed into a safe and effective treatment for lung cancer and is superior to lobectomy with thoracotomy in many regards. Development and further refinement of its technique has allowed thoracic surgeons to perform a wide variety of complex procedures in a minimally invasive fashion. With future improvement in optics, energy devices and anesthesia management, the thoracoscopic technique will continue to serve as the pillar for development of newer thoracic surgical interventions.

REFERENCES

1. Hazelrigg SR, Nunchuck SK, LoCicero J 3rd. Video assisted thoracic surgery study group data. Ann Thorac Surg 1993;56:1039–43 [discussion: 1043–44].
2. Walker WS, Codispoti M, Soon SY, et al. Long-term outcomes following VATS lobectomy for non-small cell bronchogenic carcinoma. Eur J Cardiothorac Surg 2003;23:397–402.
3. McKenna RJ Jr, Wolf RK, Brenner M, et al. Is lobectomy by video-assisted thoracic surgery an adequate cancer operation? Ann Thorac Surg 1998;66:1903–8.
4. McKenna RJ Jr. New approaches to the minimally invasive treatment of lung cancer. Cancer J 2005;11:73–6.
5. Onaitis MW, Petersen RP, Balderson SS, et al. Thoracoscopic lobectomy is a safe and versatile procedure. Ann Surg 2006;244:420–5.
6. Berry MF, D'Amico TA, Onaitis MW, et al. Thoracoscopic approach to lobectomy for lung cancer does not compromise oncologic efficacy. Ann Thorac Surg 2014;98(1):197–202.
7. D'Amico TA, Niland J, Mamet R, et al. Efficacy of mediastinal lymph node dissection during lobectomy for lung cancer by thoracoscopy and thoracotomy. Ann Thorac Surg 2011;92:226–31.
8. Cao C, Manganas C, Ang SC, et al. A meta-analysis of unmatched and matched patients comparing video-assisted thoracoscopic lobectomy and conventional open lobectomy. Ann Cardiothorac Surg 2012;1:16.
9. Yan TD, Black G, Bannon PG, et al. Systematic review and meta-analysis of randomized and nonrandomized trials on safety and efficacy of video-assisted thoracic surgery lobectomy for early-stage non-small-cell lung cancer. J Clin Oncol 2009;27:2553–62.
10. Ceppa DP, Kosinski AS, Berry MF, et al. Thoracoscopic lobectomy has increasing benefit in patients with poor pulmonary function: a Society of Thoracic Surgeons database analysis. Ann Surg 2012;256:487–93.
11. Villamizar NR, Darrabie MD, Burfeind WR, et al. Thoracoscopic lobectomy is associated with lower morbidity compared with thoracotomy. J Thorac Cardiovasc Surg 2009;138:419–25.

12. Paul S, Altorki NK, Sheng S, et al. Thoracoscopic lobectomy is associated with lower morbidity than open lobectomy: a propensity-matched analysis from the STS database. J Thorac Cardiovasc Surg 2010;139:366–78.

13. Boffa DJ, Dhamija A, Kosinski AS, et al. Fewer complications result from a video-assisted approach to anatomic resection of clinical stage I lung cancer. J Thorac Cardiovasc Surg 2014;148(2):637–43.

14. Kuritzky AM, Aswad BI, Jones RN, et al. Lobectomy by video-assisted thoracic surgery vs muscle-sparing thoracotomy for stage I lung cancer: a critical evaluation of short- and long-term outcomes. J Am Coll Surg 2015;220(6):1044–53.

15. Peterson RP, Pham D, Burfeind WR, et al. Thoracoscopic lobectomy facilitates the delivery of chemotherapy after resection for lung cancer. Ann Thorac Surg 2007; 83:1245–9.

16. Swanson SJ, Myers BF, Gunnarsson CL, et al. Video-assisted thoracoscopic lobectomy is less costly and morbid than open lobectomy: a retrospective multiinstitutional database analysis. Ann Thorac Surg 2012;93(4):1027–32.

17. Farjah F, Backhus LM, Varghese TK, et al. Ninety-day costs of video-assisted thoracic surgery versus open lobectomy for lung cancer. Ann Thorac Surg 2014;98(1):191–6.

18. Ng CS, Whelan RI, Lacy AM, et al. Is minimal access surgery for cancer associated with immunologic benefits. World J Surg 2005;29:975–81.

19. Linden PA, Bueno R, Colson YL, et al. Lung resection in patients with preoperative FEV1 < 35% predicted. Chest 2005;127(6):1984–90.

20. Santos R, Colonias A, Parda D, et al. Comparison between sublobar resection and 125Iodine brachytherapy after sublobar resection in high-risk patients with Stage I non-small-cell lung cancer. Surgery 2003;134(4):691–7 [discussion: 697].

21. Schuchert MJ, Pettiford BL, Pennathur A, et al. Anatomic segmentectomy for stage I non-small-cell lung cancer: comparison of video-assisted thoracic surgery versus open approach. J Thorac Cardiovasc Surg 2009;138(6):1318–25.

22. Berry MF, Onaitis MW, Tong BC, et al. Feasibility of hybrid thoracoscopic lobectomy and en-bloc chest wall resection. Eur J Cardiothorac Surg 2012;41(4): 888–92.

23. Agasthian T. Initial experience with video-assisted thoracoscopic bronchoplasty. Eur J Cardiothorac Surg 2013;44(4):616–23.

24. Yu D, Han Y, Zhou S, et al. Video-assisted thoracic bronchial sleeve lobectomy with bronchoplasty for treatment of lung cancer confined to a single lung lobe: a case series of Chinese patients. J Cardiothorac Surg 2014;9:67.

25. Rocco G, Martucci N, La Manna C, et al. Ten-year experience on 644 patients undergoing single-port (uniportal) video-assisted thoracoscopic surgery. Ann Thorac Surg 2013;96(2):434–8.

26. Gonzalez-Rivas D, Paradela M, Fernandez R, et al. Uniportal video-assisted thoracoscopic lobectomy: two years of experience. Ann Thorac Surg 2013;95(2): 426–32.

27. Tam JK, Lim KS. Total muscle-sparing uniportal video-assisted thoracoscopic surgery lobectomy. Ann Thorac Surg 2013;96(6):1982–6.

28. Gonzalez-Rivas D, le la Torre M, Fernandez R, et al. Video: single-incision video-assisted thoracoscopic right pneumonectomy. Surg Endosc 2012;26(7):2078–9.

29. Mcelnay PJ, Molyneux M, Krishnadas R, et al. Pain and recovery are comparable after either uniportal or multiport video-assisted thoracoscopic lobectomy: an observation study. Eur J Cardiothorac Surg 2015;47(5):912–5.

30. Zorn KC, Orvieto MA, Gong EM, et al. Robotic radical prostatectomy learning curve of a fellowship-trained laparoscopic surgeon. J Endourol 2007;21:441–7.

31. Louie BE, Farivar AS, Aye RW, et al. Early experience with robotic lung resection results in similar operative outcomes and morbidity when compared with matched video-assisted thoracoscopic surgery cases. Ann Thorac Surg 2012; 93:1598–605.

32. Park BJ. Robotic lobectomy for non-small cell lung cancer: long-term oncologic results. Thorac Surg Clin 2014;24(2):157–62.

33. Nasir BS, Bryant AS, Minnich DJ. Performing robotic lobectomy and segmentectomy: cost, profitability, and outcomes. Ann Thorac Surg 2014;98(1):203–8.

34. Kao MC, Lan CH, Huang CJ. Anesthesia for awake video-assisted thoracic surgery. Acta Anaesthesiol Taiwan 2012;50:126–30.

35. Pompeo E, Tacconi F, Mineo D, et al. The role of awake video-assisted thoracoscopic surgery in spontaneous pneumothorax. J Thorac Cardiovasc Surg 2007;133:960–6.

36. Tacconi F, Pompeo E, Fabbi E, et al. Awake video-assisted pleural decortication for empyema thoracis. Eur J Cardiothorac Surg 2010;20:594–601.

37. Chen KC, Cheng YJ, Hong MH, et al. Nonintubated thoracoscopic lung resection: a 3-year experience with 285 cases in a single institution. J Thorac Dis 2012;4(4): 347–51.

Robotic Lung Resection for Non–Small Cell Lung Cancer

Benjamin Wei, MD[a], Shady M. Eldaif, MD[b],
Robert J. Cerfolio, MD, MBA[c],*

KEYWORDS

- Robotic • Robot-assisted • Lobectomy • Lung cancer

KEY POINTS

- Robotic pulmonary lobectomy is becoming an increasingly common modality used for lung resection, and can be done with very low morbidity and mortality.
- Robotic lobectomy offers similar benefits to video-assisted thoracic surgery (VATS) lobectomy in postoperative recovery, and additional advantages in optics, dexterity, and surgeon ergonomics.
- Further comparisons between VATS and robotics in terms of ease of training, long-term oncologic efficacy, and patient outcomes are an area of active study.

INTRODUCTION

Video-assisted thoracic surgery (VATS) for pulmonary resection, including lobectomy, has become widely used among general thoracic surgeons. However, robotic surgery has certain advantages, such as 3-dimensional visualization, improved camera quality, wristed instruments, and ergonomic ease. As such, the performance of robotic-assisted pulmonary lobectomy has increased since it was first reported in the English literature in 2003.[1] Robotic surgery has certain limitations, including more complex setup time, increased costs, absence of haptic/tactile feedback, and the need for specialized equipment and training. However, results of completely portal robotic lobectomy as done with the 4-arm technique (CPRL-4) similar to or as described by

The authors have nothing to disclose.
[a] Division of Cardiothoracic Surgery, University of Alabama-Birmingham Medical Center, Birmingham, AL, USA; [b] Section of Thoracic Surgery, Northside Hospital Cancer Institute, 960 Johnson Ferry Road, Suite 100, Atlanta, GA 30342, USA; [c] Division of Cardiothoracic Surgery, University of Alabama-Birmingham Medical Center, University of Alabama at Birmingham, 703 19th Street South, ZRB 739, Birmingham, AL 352094, USA
* Corresponding author.
E-mail address: rcerfolio@uabmc.edu

Cerfolio and colleagues[2] have been shown to yield excellent results in terms of both intraoperative criteria and postoperative morbidity and mortality.

INDICATIONS

Robotic-assisted pulmonary lobectomy can be considered for any patient that is deemed fit to tolerate conventional lobectomy. In fact, patients have a better functional outcome after minimally invasive compared with open lobectomy; therefore, patients considered marginal or unfit for thoracotomy may still be considered for robotic lobectomy.[3] Burt and colleagues[4] have shown that VATS lobectomy can be performed with predicted postoperative forced expiratory volume in 1 second or diffusion capacity of the lung for carbon monoxide of less than 40% with acceptable morbidity and mortality. We believe that robotic-assisted lobectomy is similarly safe in this group of patients that had traditionally been considered inoperable.

Tumors larger than 7 cm (T3), tumors crossing fissures, and centrally located tumors may all be considered for robotic lobectomy with proper patient selection and increasing surgeon experience, but in general these factors disfavor a robotic approach. Similarly, radiologic evidence of N1 nodes, induction chemotherapy and/or radiation, calcified lymph nodes and prior thoracic surgery are not contraindications to robotic lobectomy but a robotic approach to these patients should not be selected early in one's learning curve.

Chest wall resection with robotic assistance for the parenchymal resection part of the procedure is feasible as well. VATS chest wall resection has been shown to be safe and to decrease the extent of reconstruction necessary.[5] As of yet, however, there are no published series of robotic-assisted combined lung–chest wall resections. The postoperative benefits of minimally invasive chest wall resection remain unclear.

Completely robotic sleeve lobectomy and resection with bronchoplasty have been performed at our institution, but only a single hybrid robotic–VATS case has been published from another center.[6] It is possible that the results from these operations will prove favorable; however, at this time we recommend that only practitioners with extensive experience with robotic thoracic surgery attempt these procedures. Complex vascular reconstruction remains preferentially approached from a thoracotomy.

The typical contraindications for lobectomy that apply to patients undergoing resection via thoracotomy would also apply to patients undergoing robotic lobectomy (eg, prohibitive lung function or medical comorbidities, multistation N2, gross N2 disease, or evidence of N3 disease). Patients with Pancoast tumors, tumors with extensive invasion into the mediastinum or esophagus, and those with contraindications to general anesthesia or single-lung ventilation are also poor candidates for robotic lobectomy. In addition, small nodules that are not tissue diagnosed that require lung palpation for wedge resection are considered by some as a contraindication for robotic lobectomy when a completely portal technique is used because of the inability to palpate the lung; however, lung palpation is possible with a robotic technique when a robotic-assisted technique is used. However, we have used navigational bronchoscopy with methyl blue tattooing of the nodules to help guide wedge resection or a robotic lymph node dissection and then conversion to VATS.

EQUIPMENT

The Da Vinci Surgical System is currently the only robotic system approved by the US Food and Drug Administration for lung surgery. The surgeon sits at a console some distance from the patient, who is positioned on an operating table in close proximity to the robotic unit with its 4 robotic arms. The robotic arms incorporate remote center technology, in which a fixed point in space is defined, and about it the surgical arms move so as to minimize stress on the thoracic wall during manipulations. The small proprietary Endowrist instruments attached to the arms are capable of a wide range of high-precision movements. These are controlled by the surgeon's hand movements, via "master" instruments at the console. The master instruments sense the surgeon's hand movements and translate them electronically into scaled-down micromovements to manipulate the small surgical instruments. Hand tremor is filtered out by a 6-Hz motion filter. The surgeon observes the operating field through console binoculars. The image comes from a maneuverable high-definition stereoscopic camera (endoscope) attached to one of the robot arms. The console also has foot pedals that allow the surgeon to engage and disengage different instrument arms, reposition the console master controls without the instruments themselves moving, and activate electric cautery. A second optional console allows tandem surgery and training.

PREOPERATIVE EVALUATION

Preoperative evaluation including pulmonary function testing should be obtained. Patients who are borderline in terms of overall health and/or respiratory parameters can undergo exercise testing to determine maximal oxygen consumption (Vo_2 max); patients with a Vo_2 max of greater than 15 mL/kg*min are considered moderate risk, 10 to 15 mL/kg*min are high risk, and less than 10 mL/kg*min are prohibitive risk. We routinely obtain stress testing to assess for myocardial ischemia especially in patients who have had a significant smoking history. Complete patient-specific staging should also be performed before lung resection. This includes PET-computed tomography scanning in almost all patients and the selective use of brain MRI or computed tomography (those who are symptomatic or who have large central adenocarcinomas), endobronchial ultrasound-guided fine needle aspiration, esophageal ultrasound-guided fine needle aspiration for biopsy of the posterior inferior lymph nodes and adrenals, and/or mediastinoscopy depending on the tumor size, location, radiologic findings, and institutional experience.

PORT PLACEMENT

Robotic lobectomy is a technique that can be applied to a broad range of patients and tumors. Although small, peripheral tumors in thin patients are the most easily dealt with robotically, obesity, large size of tumor, and central location of tumor are not contraindications for robotic resection.

There are several different techniques used to perform the operation. Veronesi and Melfi in 2010 reported the safety of a 4-arm robotic assisted (not completely portal) lobectomy (using a 3- to 4-cm access incision as used by VATS surgeons) in 54 patients. Ninan and Dylewski[7] in 2010 reported the effectiveness of a completely portal robotic lobectomy using 3 arms (CPRL-3) in 74 patients. Gharagozloo and colleagues[8] in 2009 reported his outcomes using a hybrid technique.

We prefer the CPRL-4 method. The technique with an SI robot is performed in the following manner for a right upper lobe. For a lower lobe the exactly same sequence is used, but the ports are placed over the ninth ribs not the eighth.

The port that is placed first is the camera port. We prefer to use a 5-mm VATS camera as opposed to the 8- or 12-mm robotic camera in case the underlying lung is injured. Once the pleural space is entered over the top of the eighth rib, warm humidified CO_2 is insufflated into the chest and a 5-mm camera is placed via the camera port and an extensive subpleural paravertebral block is carried out using 0.25% Marcaine with epinephrine from ribs 3 to 12. The next port that is, placed is the 5-mm most posterior port, which is always used for robotic arm 3; this is located 2 to 3 cm lateral to the spinous process of the vertebral bodies. As shown in **Fig. 1**, which is a right-sided resection, robotic arm 3 represents the second left hand. If you were operating in the left chest robotic, arm 3 would represent a second right-handed instrument.

The next port that is placed is robotic arm number 2, which always serves as the left hand when using an SI robot. We now currently use a 5-mm robotic DeBakey instrument or a Shertell for our left hand and used to use an 8-mm port and use a Caudierre. Once this trocar is placed only 2 trocars are left. They are carefully planned before making any incisions in the skin. The goal of these 2 trocars is to maximize the distance between the access port and the port for robotic arm 1. This affords the greatest working area for the assistant. Using a needle and injecting Marcaine into the chest, these sites are chosen by placing the access port (a 12-mm plastic disposable trocar) as low in the chest as possible and just above the diaphragmatic fibers so as not to injure it. This incision is not made until the site for robotic arm 1 is chosen as well. Note that these ports (the camera, the access port, and the site for robotic arm 1) form an isosceles triangle (see **Fig. 1**).

We use only a 0° camera to avoid injuring the intercostal nerve. Through the access port we place a 12-mm plastic port and through robotic arm 1 we use an 8-mm metal trocar and place a bipolar instrument.

For the Xi model, there are few changes in the setup. The reusable trocars come currently in 2 sizes; 8 mm is the standard size and a 12 mm, which is used for the robotic stapler. It affords easier docking technology, but one cannot use other trocar models for the robotic arm (**Fig. 2**). We begin by placing a robotic 8-mm trocar in the camera site, which could be above the eighth or ninth rib. We find that entering the chest cavity a rib space lower on the Xi affords improved visualization and also the arms can reach further on the Xi than Si so there are no downsides in placing the trocars lower when performing upper lobes. For the posterior port, an 8-mm trocar is placed and a double fenestrated tip up instrument is used in lieu of the thoracic 5-mm grasper, which is not available yet for the Xi. Finally, a 12-mm trocar is used for arm number 2 for right-sided resections or arm 3 for left-sided resections, and is used for the robotic vascular as well as thick tissue loads. There is an inner cannula that downsizes the 12-mm trocar to an 8-mm one for use of the other robotic instruments or camera "hopping" if needed. Alternately, 8-mm trocars can be used for all the robotic and camera arms if the robotic stapler is not used. The robot can come

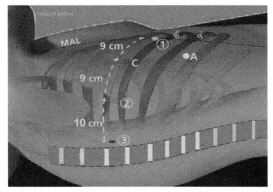

Fig. 1. Port placement for right-sided pulmonary lobectomy (CPRL-4).

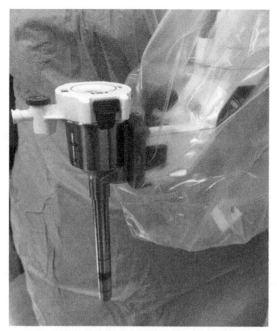

Fig. 2. New Xi trocar docking mechanism.

from the patient's sides and docked because it has a rotating boom positioned, which affords the anesthesia staff improved access to the airway (**Fig. 3**).

TECHNIQUE

After the pleural surface is inspected to confirm the absence of metastases, we proceed with mediastinal lymph node dissection.

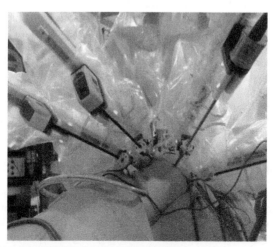

Fig. 3. Robotic Xi boom positioned over patient body.

Right Side

The inferior pulmonary ligament is divided to get to lymph node station 9. It is removed along with lymph node station 8. Robotic arm 3 is used to retract the lower lobe medially and anteriorly to remove lymph nodes from station 7. Care is taken to control the 2 feeding arteries that make the subcarinal lymph node bloody. Robotic arm 3 is used to retract the upper lobe inferiorly and robotic arms 1 and 2 are used to dissect out stations 2R and 4R, clearing the space between the superior vena cava anteriorly, the esophagus posteriorly, and the azygos vein inferiorly. Avoiding dissection too far superiorly can prevent injury to the right recurrent laryngeal nerve that wraps around the subclavian artery.

Left Side

The inferior pulmonary ligament is divided to facilitate the removal of lymph node station 9. The nodes in station 8 are then removed. Station 7 is accessed in the space between the inferior pulmonary vein and lower lobe bronchus, lateral to the esophagus. If still in position, the lower lobe is retracted medially/anteriorly with robotic arm 3 during this process. Absence of the lower lobe facilitates dissection of level 7 from the left. Finally, robotic arm 3 is used to wrap around the left upper lobe and press it inferiorly to allow dissection of stations 5 and 6. Care should be taken while working in the aortopulmonary window to avoid injury to the left recurrent laryngeal nerve. Station 2L cannot typically be accessed during left sided mediastinal lymph node dissection owing to the presence of the aortic arch, but the 4L node is commonly removed.

Once the absence of mediastinal lymph node metastases is confirmed, we then proceed with pulmonary lobectomy. In situations where a confirmatory preoperative biopsy has not been done and the tumor is peripheral, a wedge resection may be done to establish a definitive diagnosis of a cancer before going ahead with lobectomy.

The order of structures to be isolated and divided is not always the same; however, certain patterns emerge depending on the lobe to be removed. A few principles, however, are worth keeping in mind:

- Lymph nodes in interlobar and intersegmental lesions are removed first to facilitate dissection of the vascular structures and bronchi.
- Bipolar cautery may be used to dissect the fissure with minimal air leak. As opposed to VATS, which generally emphasizes stapling of the fissure as one of the last steps of lobectomy, for robotic lobectomies the fissure is often approached first so that vascular structures can be identified and isolated.
- It is helpful to encircle the structures to be divided with vessel loops before attempting to pass the stapler. The stapler should be passed through the port that offers the best angle of attack, whether it is robot arm #1, #2, or the assistant port. If using a robot port, the port itself will have to be removed before putting the stapler through.

WEDGE RESECTION

Wedge resection of a nodule may be necessary to confirm the presence of cancer before proceeding with lobectomy. Because the current iteration of the robot does not offer tactile feedback, special techniques may be necessary to identify a nodule that is not obvious on visual inspection. An empty ring forceps may be used via the assistant port to palpate the nodule. Alternatively, preoperative marking of the nodule with a dye marker injected via navigational bronchoscopy can facilitate location of the nodule. Preoperative confirmation of a cancer diagnosis with tissue biopsy is helpful to avoid being unable to locate the nodule intraoperatively.

THE 5 LOBECTOMIES

A certain degree of adaptability is necessary for performance of robotic lobectomy. Structures may be isolated and divided in the order that the patient's individual anatomy permits. What follows is a description of an outline of the typical conduct of each lobectomy.

Right Upper Lobectomy

- Retraction of the right upper lobe laterally and posteriorly with robot arm 3 helps to expose the hilum.
- The bifurcation between the right upper and middle lobar veins is developed by dissecting it off the underlying pulmonary artery.
- The 10R lymph node between the truncus branch and the superior pulmonary vein should be removed or swept up toward the lung, which exposes the truncus branch.
- The superior pulmonary vein is encircled with the vessel loop and then divided (**Figs. 4** and **5**). The truncus branch is then divided.
- The right upper lobe is then reflected anteriorly to expose the bifurcation of the right main stem bronchus. There is usually a lymph node here that should be dissected out to expose the bifurcation. The right upper lobe bronchus is then encircled and divided. Care must be taken to apply only minimal retraction on the specimen to avoid tearing the remaining pulmonary artery branches.
- Finally, the posterior segmental artery to the right upper lobe is exposed, the surrounding N1 nodes removed, and the artery encircled and divided (**Fig. 6**).
- The upper lobe is reflected again posteriorly, and the anterior aspect of the pulmonary artery is inspected to make sure that there are no arterial branches remaining. If not, then the fissure between the upper and middle lobes, and the upper and lower lobes, is then divided. This is typically done from anterior to posterior, but may be done in the reverse direction if the space between the pulmonary artery and right middle lobe is already developed. During completion of the

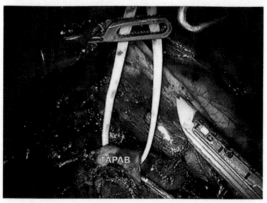

Fig. 4. The truncus arterial branch (TAPAB) with vessel loop around it for staple guidance.

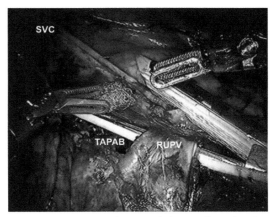

Fig. 5. Stapler positioning around the right upper lobe vein branches (RULV) off of the right superior pulmonary vein. Truncus branch (TAPAB) labeled and superior vena cava (SVC) in the left upper corer.

fissure, the right upper lobe should be lifted up to ensure that the specimen bronchus is included in the specimen.

Right Middle Lobectomy

- Retraction of the right middle lobe laterally and posteriorly with robot arm I helps to expose the hilum.
- The bifurcation between the right upper and middle lobar veins is developed by dissecting it off the underlying pulmonary artery. The right middle lobe vein is encircled and divided.
- The fissure between the right middle and lower lobes, if not complete, is divided from anterior to posterior. Care should be taken to avoid transecting segmental arteries to the right lower lobe.
- The right middle lobe bronchus is then isolated. It will be running from left to right in the fissure. Level 11 lymph nodes are dissected from around it. It is encircled

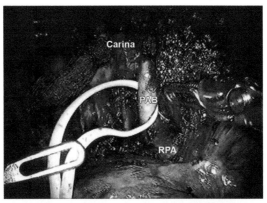

Fig. 6. Dissecting in the fissure to expose the posterior ascending branch (PAB) from the right pulmonary artery (RPA). The carina is viewed in the background.

and divided, taking care to avoid injuring the right middle lobar artery that is located directly behind it.
- Dissection of the fissure should continue posteriorly until the branches to the superior segment are identified. Then the 1 or 2 right middle lobar segmental arteries are isolated and divided (**Fig. 7**).
- Stapling of middle lobar structures may be facilitated by passing the stapler from posterior to anterior, to have a greater working distance.
- The fissure between right middle and upper lobes is then divided.

Right Lower Lobectomy

- The inferior pulmonary ligament should be divided to the level of the inferior pulmonary vein.
- The bifurcation of the right superior and inferior pulmonary veins should be dissected out. The location of the right middle lobar vein should be positively identified to avoid inadvertent transection.
- A subadventitial plane on the ongoing pulmonary artery should be established. If the major fissure is not complete, then it should be divided. The superior segmental artery and the right middle lobe arterial branches are identified. The superior segmental artery is isolated and divided. The common trunk to right lower lobe basilar segments may be taken as long as this does not compromise the middle lobar segmental artery/arteries; otherwise, dissection may have to extend further distally to ensure safe division (**Fig. 8**).
- The inferior pulmonary vein is divided.
- The right lower lobe bronchus is isolated, taking care to visualize the right middle lobar bronchus crossing from left to right. The surrounding lymph nodes, as usual, are dissected and the bronchus divided (**Fig. 9**). If there is any question of compromising the right middle lobe bronchus, the surgeon can ask the anesthesiologist to hand ventilate the right lung to confirm that the middle lobe expands.

Left Upper Lobectomy

- Retraction of the left upper lobe laterally and posteriorly with robot arm 3 helps to expose the hilum.

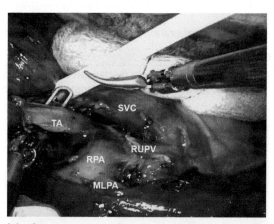

Fig. 7. Dissection of the fissure anteriorly showing the middle lobe pa branch (MLPA) off the right pulmonary artery (RPA) and the truncus branch (TA) as well. The superior vena cava (SVC) appears at the top of the image and an already ligated right upper lobe vein (RUPV) staple line is labeled.

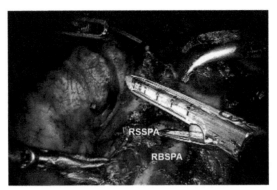

Fig. 8. Fissure dissection exposing the right superior segmental pa branch (RSSPA) and the right basilar segmental trunk (RBSPA).

- The presence of both superior and inferior pulmonary veins is confirmed, and the bifurcation dissected.
- The lung is then reflected anteriorly with robotic arm 3 and interlobar dissection is started, going from posterior to anterior.
- If the fissure is not complete, then it will need to be divided. Reflecting the lung posteriorly again and establishing a subadventitial plane will be helpful. The branches to the lingula are encountered and divided in the fissure during this process. The posterior segmental artery is also isolated and divided (**Figs. 10 and 11**). Division of the lingular artery or arteries can be done before or after division of the posterior segmental artery.
- The superior pulmonary vein is isolated then divided (**Fig. 12**). Because the superior pulmonary vein can be fairly wide, it may require that the lingular and upper division branches be transected separately.
- Often the next structure that can be divided readily will be the left upper lobar bronchus, as opposed to the anterior and apical arterial branches to the left upper lobe. The upper lobe bronchus should be encircled and divided, often passing the stapler from robotic arm 1 to avoid injuring the main pulmonary artery (**Fig. 13**).
- Finally, the remaining arterial branches are encircled and divided.

Left Lower Lobectomy

- The inferior pulmonary ligament should be divided to the level of the inferior pulmonary vein. The lower lobe is then reflected posteriorly by robotic arm 3.

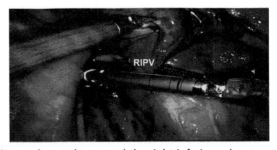

Fig. 9. The robotic vascular stapler around the right inferior pulmonary vein (RIPV).

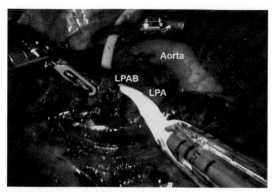

Fig. 10. The apical pulmonary artery branch (LPAB) is circumferentially dissected of the main left pulmonary artery (LPA) with the descending aorta in the background. Note the complete AP window lymph node dissection exposing the vagus nerve and the left recurrent laryngeal nerve (not labeled).

- The bifurcation of the left superior and inferior pulmonary veins should be dissected out.
- The lung is reflected anteriorly by robotic arm 3. The superior segmental artery is identified. The posterior ascending arteries to the left upper lobe are frequently visible from this view also. The superior segmental artery is isolated and divided. The common trunk to left lower lobe basilar segments may be taken as long as this does not compromise the middle lobar segmental artery/arteries; otherwise, dissection may have to extend further distally to ensure safe division. If the fissure is not complete, this will need to be divided to expose the ongoing pulmonary artery to the lower lobe.
- After division of the arterial branches, the lung is reflected again posteriorly. The inferior pulmonary vein is divided.
- The left lower lobe bronchus is isolated. The surrounding lymph nodes, as usual, are dissected and the bronchus divided.
- For left lower lobectomy, it may be simpler to wait until after resection is performed before targeting the subcarinal space for removal of level 7 lymph nodes.

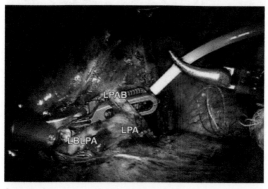

Fig. 11. Complete fissure dissection of the left pulmonary artery (LPA) showing accessory posterior pa branch (LPAB) and lingular branch (LBLPA).

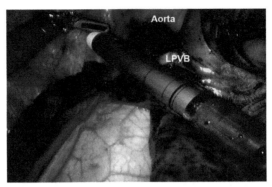

Fig. 12. The robotic vascular stapler around the apical branch (LPVB) of the left superior pulmonary vein. The distal arch of the aorta appears at the top of the image.

AVOIDANCE OF INTRAOPERATIVE COMPLICATIONS/TROUBLESHOOTING

Intraoperative complications can be minimized and managed by following certain rules and guidelines.

- The passing of vascular staplers around fragile structure such as the pulmonary artery and/or vein deserves special attention. Carefully orchestrated moves and clear communication is needed between the bedside assistant and the surgeon. We have developed our own communication system between the bedside assistant and the surgeon to prevent iatrogenic injuries. This uses the anvil of the stapler as the hour hand of a clock and the degree of articulation is also quantified and communicated.
- Robotic instruments should be initially inserted under direct vision during thoracic surgery for their initial placement. Once safely positioned, instruments then can be quickly and safely inserted or changed for other instruments by properly using the memory feature of the robot that automatically inserts any new instruments to a position that is exactly 1 cm proximal to its latest position. However, if this feature is used, it is incumbent on the surgeon to ensure that

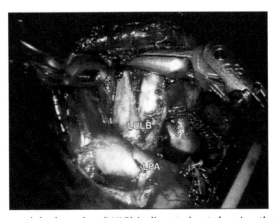

Fig. 13. The left upper lobe bronchus (LULB) is dissected out showing the trisegmental and lingular divisions with the left pa (LPA) caudad to it.

no vital structure have moved into the path of that newly placed instrument. The most common structure would be the lung.

- A rolled-up sponge should always be immediately accessible when working around vascular structures. If an injury occurs, the first step should be to tamponade the structure with the sponge. A minor injury may respond to this packing alone. If bleeding is massive or persists, a thoracotomy will be necessary. Lap pads should be inserted via the assistant port and packed around the injury to control bleeding. The robot is then dedocked and a thoracotomy made.
- The "drop zone" for the specimen should be well away from the pulmonary artery, which can be injured during this process if care is not taken.
- To remove the specimen, the assistant nonrobotic port is enlarged posteriorly to avoid injuring the diagram.
- The robotic arms are removed under direct vision with insufflation discontinued to confirm the absence of bleeding.

Table 1 shows how to trouble shoot common problems encountered during robotic lobectomy.

RESULTS
Perioperative Morbidity/Mortality

Robotic lobectomy can be done with very low morbidity and mortality. We have previously demonstrated a 30-day mortality rate of 0.25%, a 90-day mortality rate of 0.5%, and a major morbidity rate of 9.6% in patients undergoing robotic anatomic pulmonary resection (lobectomy and segmentectomy).[9] Robotic lobectomy is associated with decreased rates of blood loss, blood transfusion, air leak, chest tube duration, length of stay, and mortality compared with thoracotomy.[10,11] With experience, conversion rates of less than 1% to thoracotomy may be achieved, although 3% to 5% is more typically reported.[2,10]

Oncologic Efficacy

Park and colleagues[12] showed that the survival of patients undergoing robotic lobectomy to be similar to historical survival data from VATS and open lobectomy series. This multiinstitutional study of 325 patients was characterized by a median follow-up of 27 months, and demonstrated a 5-year survival rate of 80% overall (91% for stage IA, 88% for stage IB, 49% for stage II). The 3-year survival for patients with stage IIIA disease was 43%. Although it is reasonable to hypothesize that robotic lobectomy will demonstrate at least equivalent results to VATS and open lobectomy from an oncologic perspective, more study is needed before this conclusion can be reached.

Lymph Node Dissection

Lymph node dissection with the robot is facilitated by the utilization of wristed instruments and the presence of bipolar cautery on dissectors. Most practitioners of robotic lobectomy perform a dissection of the fissure, with corresponding lymph node resection, although many VATS surgeons perform a "fissureless" technique that may lead to lymph nodes being incorporated in the specimen rather than individually dissected. One study demonstrated that upstaging of early stage lung cancers by robotic lobectomy (clinical T1a, T1b, and T2a) occurred in 10.9% of patients; 6.6% were upstaged owing to hilar (pN1) disease and 4.3% were upstaged owing to mediastinal (pN2) disease. Compared with prior series, this rate of overall nodal upstaging was similar to VATS (8%–12%), but lower than thoracotomy (20%–25%).[13] Other investigators have demonstrated a comparable number of lymph nodes dissected during robotic

Table 1 Troubleshooting of common problems during robotic lobectomy	
Problems	**Solutions**
Robotic arms are not responding to hand movement	1. Ensure trocar's remote center is in chest. 2. Ensure trocar's docked properly to robotic arms. 3. Ensure sterile plastic gown covering robotic arms is not interfering with wheeled mechanism of robot. 4. Ensure surgeons' hand not maximized at console.
The camera is fogging	1. Place humidified CO_2 insufflation through non access port (and not through the camera port). 2. Preheat the camera. 3. Evacuate smoke from the intraoperative field.
There are conflicts between robotic arms 3 and 1 or 2	1. Ensure $\geq$10 cm between robotic arm 3 and closest robotic arm (robotic arm 1 or 2). 2. Use a 5-mm thoracic lung grasper as the instrument of choice through the most posterior robotic arm. 3. After docking, ensure the link 2's of robotic arms are aligned parallel to one another. 4. When surgeon toggles between robotic arm 3 and 2 or 1, ensure the nonactive instrument is placed anteriorly toward chest wall.
The bipolar cautery or thoracic dissector is not working.	Ensure the bipolar... 1. ...source is connected to robot, 2. ...energy source is functioning, and 3. ...cord is not damaged.
There is a sudden loss of working space	1. Ensure DLET is properly positioned. 2. Inflate more air in bronchial cuff. 3. Ensure no leaks out of ports if using a completely portal technique. 4. Ensure all valves are closed on ports. 5. Do not place sucker in chest on suction unless immersed under water or blood.
You are unable to achieve proper angle of stapler to come across vessels or fissures	1. Try placing stapler through robotic access port or robotic arm 1 or 2 to achieve best angle. 2. Use a stapler which maximizes the degrees of rotation and articulation. 3. Do not force the stapler; tie vessels with suture or use an 8-mm robotic clips on vessel.
There is difficulty in bagging specimen	1. Use a bag that provides easy opening and closing by bedside assistant. 2. Place bag under trocar before deployment. 3. Place bag in the most anterior superior aspect of chest to maximize use of gravity, space and keep bag away from stapled hilar structures. 4. Use robotic arm 3 to place specimen into bag and then hold back of the bag in place while stuffing specimen into bag with robotic arms 1 and 2.

Abbreviation: DLET, double lumen endotracheal tube.

and VATS lobectomy.[14] Nodal upstaging rates from VATS versus robotic lobectomy have also been shown to be similar in patients with clinical N0 lung cancer (15.2% vs 13.2%; $P = .72$).[15] It is not clear yet whether or not use of the robot for lobectomy will allow surgeons to achieve an equivalent nodal dissection to thoracotomy.

Table 2
Results reported in series of robotic-assisted lobectomies

Author, Year	n	Conversion Rate (%)	Morbidity (%)	Perioperative Mortality (%)	Median LOS (d)	Other Notes
Cerfolio et al,[2] 2011	168	7.7	27	0	2	Decreased morbidity, improved QOL, shorter LOS than open lobectomy
Park et al,[19] 2006	30	12	26	0	4.5	—
Veronesi et al,[20] 2009	54	13	20	0	4.5	Shorter LOS than open lobectomy
Gharagozloo et al,[8] 2009	100	—	21	3	4	—

Abbreviations: LOS, length of stay; QOL, quality of life.

Cost

Shorter length of stay and decreased morbidity translate into lower hospital costs, and therefore generally favor minimally invasive pulmonary resection over pulmonary resection via thoracotomy. Robotic lobectomy has been shown to have decreased cost compared with open lobectomy.[9] However, the price of a DaVinci SI Surgical System is $1.7 million, and the price of a second console is $450,000. The maintenance cost per year per robot is estimated at $140,000, and the replacement costs for the instruments that are limited in terms of reusability are significant.[16] When compared with VATS lobectomy, robotic pulmonary lobectomy has a higher overall hospital cost, ranging from an additional $3000 to $5000 per case.[17,18] Nevertheless, robotic lobectomy continues to be a profitable endeavor for hospital systems, with an estimated median profit margin of around $3500 per patient.[9]

SUMMARY

Robotic pulmonary lobectomy is becoming an increasingly common modality used for lung resection, and can be done with very low morbidity and mortality, as we and other investigators have demonstrated (**Table 2**). Robotic lobectomy is advantageous when compared with open lobectomy with regards to short-term outcomes, both in community and academic settings.[10,11] The modality offers many of the same benefits in terms of perioperative morbidity and mortality that VATS lobectomy, with some additional advantages in terms of optics, dexterity, and surgeon ergonomics. Clearly, robotic assistance can be a safe and useful technology for lung resection when surgeons are properly trained. Further comparisons between VATS and robotics in terms of ease of training, long-term oncologic efficacy, and patient outcomes are an area of active study.

REFERENCES

1. Morgan JA, Ginsburg ME, Sonett JR, et al. Advanced thoracoscopic procedures are facilitated by computer-aided robotic technology. Eur J Cardiothorac Surg 2003;23:883–7.

2. Cerfolio RJ, Bryant AS, Skylizard L, et al. Initial consecutive experience of completely portal robotic pulmonary resection with 4 arms. J Thorac Cardiovasc Surg 2011;142:740–6.

3. Handy JR, Asaph JW, Douville EC. Does video-assisted thoracoscopic lobectomy for lung cancer provide improved functional outcomes compared with open lobectomy? Eur J Cardiothorac Surg 2010;37:451–5.

4. Burt BM, Kosinski AS, Shrager JB, et al. Thoracoscopic lobectomy is associated with acceptable morbidity and mortality in patients with predicted postoperative forced expiratory volume in 1 second or diffusing capacity for carbon monoxide less than 40% of normal. J Thorac Cardiovasc Surg 2014;148:19–28.

5. Hennon MW, Dexter EU, Huang M, et al. Does thoracoscopic surgery decrease the morbidity of combined lung and chest wall resection? Ann Thorac Surg 2015;99:1929–34.

6. Schmid T, Augustin F, Kainz G, et al. Hybrid video-assisted thoracic surgery-robotic minimally invasive right upper lobe sleeve lobectomy. Ann Thorac Surg 2011;91:1961–5.

7. Ninan M, Dylewski MR. Total port-access robot assisted pulmonary lobectomy without utility thoracotomy. Eur J Cardiothorac Surg 2010;38:231–2.

8. Gharagozloo F, Margolis M, Tempesta B, et al. Robot-assisted lobectomy for early-stage lung cancer: report of 100 consecutive cases. Ann Thorac Surg 2009;88:380–4.

9. Park BJ, Flores RM. Cost comparison of robotic, video-assisted thoracic surgery and thoracotomy approaches to pulmonary lobectomy. Thorac Surg Clin 2008; 18:297–300.

10. Adams RD, Bolton WD, Stephenson JE, et al. Initial multicenter community robotic lobectomy experience: comparisons to a national database. Ann Thorac Surg 2014;97:1893–8.

11. Kent M, Want T, Whyte R, et al. Open, video-assisted thoracic surgery, and robotic lobectomy: review of a national database. Ann Thorac Surg 2014;97: 236–42.

12. Park BJ, Melfi F, Mussi A, et al. Robotic lobectomy for non-small cell lung cancer (NSCLC): long-term oncologic results. J Thorac Cardiovasc Surg 2012;143: 383–9.

13. Wilson JL, Louie BE, Cerfolio RJ, et al. The prevalence of nodal upstaging during robotic lung resection in early stage non-small cell lung cancer. Ann Thorac Surg 2014;97:1901–7.

14. Hs Lee, Jang HJ. Thoracoscopic mediastinal lymph node dissection for lung cancer. Semin Thorac Cardiovasc Surg 2012;24:131–41.

15. Lee B, Shapiro M, Rutledge JR, et al. Nodal upstaging in robotic and video assisted lobectomy for clinical N0 lung cancer. Ann Thorac Surg 2015;100:229–33.

16. Nasir BS, Bryant AS, Minnich DJ, et al. Performing robotic lobectomy and segmentectomy: cost, profitability, and outcomes. Ann Thorac Surg 2014;98:203–8.

17. Deen SA, Wilson JL, Wishire CL, et al. Defining the cost of care for lobectomy and segmentectomy: a comparison of open, video-assisted thoracoscopic, and robotic approaches. Ann Thorac Surg 2014;97:1000–7.

18. Swanson SJ, Miller DL, McKenna RJ, et al. Comparing robot-assisted thoracic surgical lobectomy with conventional video-assisted thoracic surgical lobectomy and wedge resection: results from a multihospital database. J Thorac Cardiovasc Surg 2014;147:929–37.

19. Park BJ, Flores RM, Rusch VW. Robotic assistance for video-assisted thoracic surgical lobectomy: technique and initial results. J Thorac Cardiovasc Surg 2006;131:54–9.
20. Veronesis G, Galetta D, Maisonneuve P, et al. Four-arm robotic lobectomy for the treatment of early-stage lung cancer. J Thorac Cardiovasc Surg 2010;140:19–25.

Pneumonectomy for Non–Small Cell Lung Cancer

David J. Sugarbaker, MD[a],*, Ricky J. Haywood-Watson, MD, PhD[b],
Ori Wald, MD, PhD[c]

KEYWORDS

- Pneumonectomy • Multimodal therapy • Operative technique • Lung cancer
- Preoperative evaluation • Operative complications

KEY POINTS

- The diagnosis and management of lung cancer requires a multimodal approach that often involves surgical resection.
- Accurate preoperative staging is essential in selecting patients who would benefit the most from pneumonectomy.
- Pneumonectomy is usually indicated when tumors are centrally located, involving the hilum, or as part of a multimodal approach to locally advanced tumors.
- Pneumonectomy is a difficult and technically demanding operation associated with a high rate of perioperative morbidity.

INTRODUCTION

Lung cancer remains the most common cancer in the world, both in terms of new cases (1.8 million cases, 12.9% of total) and deaths (1.6 million deaths, 19.4).[1–3] The 2 major histologic types of lung cancer are small cell lung cancer (SCLC) and non–SCLC (NSCLC). SCLC accounts for 20% of all new lung cancer diagnoses.[2] Although SCLC is the more aggressive cancer, limited stage SCLC is usually responsive to systemic chemotherapy, with median survival rates of 18 to 36 months and 5-year survival of 20% to 25%.[4] In contrast, NSCLC accounts for 80% of all new lung cancers and is amenable to surgical excision in select patients. NSCLC

The authors have nothing to disclose.
[a] Division of General Thoracic Surgery, Michael E. DeBakey Department of General Surgery, Lung Institute, Baylor College of Medicine, One Baylor Plaza MS390, Houston, TX 77030, USA; [b] Michael E. DeBakey Department of General Surgery, Baylor College of Medicine, One Baylor Plaza MS390, Houston, TX 77030, USA; [c] Division of General Thoracic Surgery, Michael E. DeBakey Department of General Surgery, Baylor College of Medicine, One Baylor Plaza MS390, Houston, TX 77030, USA
* Corresponding author.
E-mail address: david.sugarbaker@bcm.edu

Surg Oncol Clin N Am 25 (2016) 533–551
http://dx.doi.org/10.1016/j.soc.2016.02.012
1055-3207/16/$ – see front matter © 2016 Elsevier Inc. All rights reserved.

includes three major subtypes; squamous cell carcinoma (30%-40%), adenocarcinoma (25%-30%), and large cell lung carcinoma (<10%).[5]

A multidisciplinary approach to the diagnosis and management of lung cancer is essential to design a personalized treatment plan for each patient. The overall clinical status of the patient, pathologic subtype, and disease stage are all taken into account when designing the treatment plan.[6–10] Staging is specifically important because the anatomic extent of the tumor has a significant impact on the treatment of choice and the final prognosis.[11] Original staging classifications were based on the TNM system dating back to 1944 and the multiple revisions of the staging classifications that have taken place since then.[3] The most recent edition (seventh edition) of the lung cancer staging system has been defined by the International Association for the Study of Lung Cancer using a patient database of more than 100,000 patients. The next revision of the lung cancer staging system is slated to be published in 2016.[3]

Early and intermediate stage cancers (I and II) have in common the fact that a complete resection is achieved by anatomic resection, either lobectomy or pneumonectomy.[12] Locally advanced lung cancers (IIIA and IIIB) are also amenable to surgical resection in select groups using a multimodal approach to therapy.[13–15] Pneumonectomy for non–SCLC is usually indicated when tumors are located centrally and invading vascular structures or the proximal bronchus, or when part of a multimodal approach to locally advanced tumors. Pneumonectomy, when part of a multimodal approach, has been shown to offer improved encouraging long term survival rates in selected patients with N2 disease.[13,15–19]

Neoadjuvant chemotherapy and radiation are not recommended as treatment options for early to intermediate stage lung cancer.[7,12] However, neoadjuvant chemoradiation has been shown as an effective tool to achieve regression of N2 nodes.[20] Adjuvant chemotherapy is recommended for stage IIA, IIB, and IIIA cancers, whereas adjuvant radiation therapy is currently only recommended for patients with N2 nodal disease to decrease local recurrence.[7,12,21] Current data describe 5-year survival rates for stages I and II as 60% to 80% and 30% to 50%, respectively.[8,22] The 5-year survival for stage III disease has been reported to be approximately 25% to 45% when using a multimodal approach to therapy.[12,14,23–25] Accurate preoperative staging is essential in selecting patients who would benefit the most from a multidisciplinary approach to treatment of locally advanced disease that includes pneumonectomy.[26,27]

PREOPERATIVE WORKUP
Staging

First, a complete history and a physical examination that focuses on performance status and weight loss as well as on identification of chest wall and lymph node involvement, and on sings of distant spread is performed. Next, a computed tomography scan of the chest and a PET/computed tomography scan are performed.[28–30] These measures will rule out distant metastases, other than brain metastases. Patients without symptoms of headache and with a PET-negative mediastinum are unlikely to have brain metastases, so brain computed tomography scans or MRIs are not mandatory for preoperative staging. However, brain imaging should be included in the standard workup of those patients with locally advanced disease (stage IIIA or IIIB) or preoperative evaluation suggesting a high likelihood of nodal involvement to rule out brain metastases.

All patients with lung cancer should first undergo preoperative staging (**Box 1**). Candidates for pneumonectomy typically have large or central tumors and thus are likely

---

Box 1
Preoperative evaluation of potential pneumonectomy patients

1. Complete history and a physical examination with focuses on performance status, weight loss, detection of chest wall involvement and detection of lymphatic or distant metastatic spread.

2. Imaging
   a. Chest computed tomography scan
   b. PET scan with or without brain MRI

3. Invasive Diagnostic Procedures
   a. Mediastinoscopy/endobronchial ultrasound with transbronchial needle aspiration
   b. Thoracoscopy

---

to have mediastinal metastases. PET scans are relatively sensitive for detecting mediastinal metastases; nevertheless, they are still not as accurate as mediastinoscopy and newer minimally invasive techniques for tissue acquisition like endobronchial ultrasound with transbronchial needle aspiration.[31–34] Thus, we believe that tissue biopsy (either with endobronchial ultrasound, preoperative mediastinoscopy, or thoracoscopy), is indicated for patients who may undergo pneumonectomy, even if they have a PET-negative mediastinum.

Surgical Evaluation

Having mentioned the importance of surgical staging of the mediastinum, 2 other surgical evaluations should be considered in the preoperative workup of a pneumonectomy patient. Bronchoscopic evaluation of the airway will ensure that a patient with a hilar mass does not also have a contralateral endobronchial lesion. In the event the surgery is successful, a pneumonectomy would subject the patient to a difficult and possibly lengthy recovery with no impact on overall survival.[35] Thoracoscopic evaluation and staging of the pleural space has the potential to benefit patients undergoing pneumonectomy in multiple ways.[36] Thoracoscopy helps to identify pleural metastases that cannot be identified by conventional imaging techniques. Thoracoscopic nodal sampling or lymphadenectomy can evaluate suspicious nodes in patients who have not had tissue sampling and can also facilitate the sampling of nodes that are inaccessible to other biopsy techniques. Thoracoscopy can be used for surgical planning to determine the incision used for resection.

Cardiopulmonary Evaluation

Preoperative lung function is another valuable data point in the workup of a pneumonectomy patient. Patients with a preoperative forced expiratory volume in 1 second (FEV_1) of more than 2 L are considered eligible for pneumonectomy. For patients with a low or borderline FEV_1 it is useful to calculate the predicted postoperative lung function and diffusing capacity of the lung for carbon monoxide because these parameters were shown to correlate with postoperative complications after pneumonectomy.[37–39] Patients with a predicted postoperative FEV_1 of more than 800 mL have been shown to have adequate pulmonary reserve to undergo resection in long-term follow-up.[40] Most patients requiring a pneumonectomy have obstructing cancers and are thus compensating for the loss of substantial lung function in the affected lung by depending primarily on the unaffected lung for respiration. Quantitative perfusion scanning (V/Q scan) has been used for more than 30 years to determine the relative contribution of each lung to the patient's total lung function and can be valuable when interpreting preoperative lung function studies.[41,42] Cardiac evaluations (ie, echocardiography, stress testing) and preoperative referral to a cardiologist should be performed in all patients. We routinely perform echocardiograms in patients with locally advanced disease to evaluate overall cardiac function and to assess any possible tumor invasion of the pericardium. Lower extremity duplex Doppler ultrasound to rule out deep venous thrombosis should also be considered in patients with locally advanced disease (**Box 2**).

TECHNIQUE
Left Pneumonectomy

While in the preoperative holding area, the anesthesia team places an epidural catheter for postoperative pain management. The patient is first positioned supine and intubated with a single lumen endotracheal tube and a bronchial blocker passed into the lung to be removed. Alternatively, a double lumen endotracheal tube, or the endotracheal tube can be purposefully main-stemmed in the bronchus of the lung to be preserved. To optimize the hemodynamic monitoring of the patient we routinely place a urinary catheter, an arterial line and a Swan–Ganz catheter. Once the anesthesiology team is ready, the patient is repositioned in the right or left lateral decubitus position. The lung on the side to be resected is occluded and positioning of the tube and blocker confirmed.

A muscle-sparing posterolateral thoracotomy skin incision is made. The latissimus dorsi muscle is divided and the serratus anterior muscle is retracted superiorly. The pleural space is approached via the fifth intercostal space (**Fig. 1**). Chest spreaders are placed to facilitate exposure. If needed the rib can be transected posteriorly. The chest is inspected for pleural effusion and the chest wall and lung are assessed for metastatic spread. Any suspicious tissue is sent for frozen section analysis. Next, the mediastinal pleura and inferior pulmonary ligament is divided circumferentially around the hilum using either scissors or electrocautery. Harvesting the lymph nodes in the aortopulmonary window gives better exposure to the proximal pulmonary artery. This technique must be performed carefully to avoid injuring the recurrent laryngeal nerve, which branches off the vagus nerve on the inferior surface of the aortic arch and then dives into the mediastinum immediately inferior and adherent to the arch (**Fig. 2**). The phrenic nerve should also be preserved, unless it is involved in the tumor. The phrenic nerve is at risk because it may abut the anterior aspect of the nodes in the anteroposterior window. Sometimes the vagus superior to the aorta or the recurrent nerve must be harvested if either is involved with the tumor. However, resection of these nerves will lead to vocal cord paralysis. Harvesting

---

Box 2
Preoperative evaluation of cardiopulmonary status before pneumonectomy

1. Complete pulmonary function testing with spirometry and diffusing capacity of the lung for carbon monoxide.

2. Quantitative perfusion scanning to evaluate lung function on each side.

3. Calculation of predicted postoperative forced expiratory volume in 1 second and diffusing capacity of the lung for carbon monoxide. Maximum oxygen consumption by exercise stress test.

4. Echocardiography.

5. Evaluation by cardiologist with or without referral for additional tests (stress test, stress echocardiography, left and right heart catheterization).

6. Lower extremity duplex Doppler ultrasound examination.

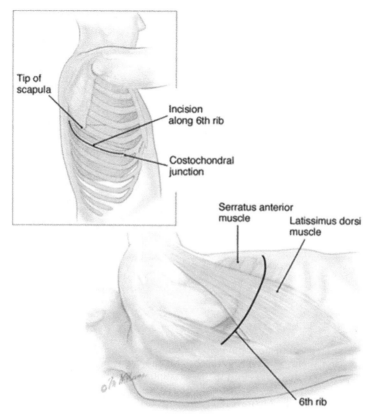

Fig. 1. A muscle-sparing posterolateral thoracotomy skin incision is made. The latissimus dorsi muscle is divided and the serratus anterior muscle is retracted superiorly. (*From* Sugarbaker DJ, Bueno R, Colson YL, et al, editors. Adult Chest Surgery. 2nd edition. New York: The McGraw-Hill Company; 2015; with permission.)

the subcarinal lymph nodes provides better exposure of the bronchus and also allows better palpation of the bronchus. Once the hilum of the lung is free, the pulmonary artery is dissected away from the superior pulmonary vein anteroinferiorly and the bronchus posteriorly (**Figs. 3** and **4**). In most instances, this can be done bluntly, before mobilization or division of the superior vein. Dissecting and dividing the vein first is an alternative in patients with inferiorly positioned artery or superiorly positioned vein.

The pulmonary artery should be occluded before its division to ensure that pneumonectomy will not cause right ventricular failure or pulmonary hypertension. Communication with the anesthesiologist is imperative after the artery is clamped to assess the systolic blood pressure and oxygenation and determine if the patient will tolerate pneumonectomy. If hemodynamic instability or hypoxia develops, the pulmonary artery catheter can be used to direct inotropic therapy, but in most cases, it is necessary to abandon the procedure altogether. Care should be taken during this maneuver not to "fracture" the pulmonary artery when temporarily occluding the vessel. (Digital occlusion may be preferable in this situation.)

Additional pulmonary artery length (to allow complete resection) can be obtained by using 1 or both of 2 maneuvers: dividing the ligamentum arteriosum while paying

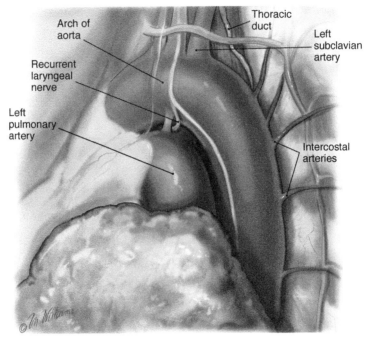

Fig. 2. When dissecting out aortopulmonary nodes, care must be taken to avoid injuring the recurrent laryngeal nerve, which branches off the vagus nerve on the inferior surface of the aortic arch and then dives into the mediastinum immediately inferior and adherent to the arch. (*From* Sugarbaker DJ, Bueno R, Colson YL, et al, editors. Adult Chest Surgery. 2nd edition. New York: The McGraw-Hill Company; 2015; with permission.)

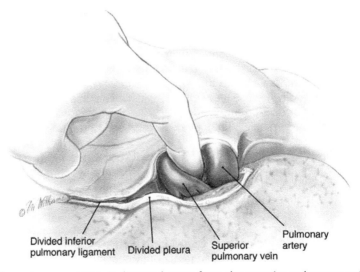

Fig. 3. The pulmonary artery is dissected away from the superior pulmonary vein. (*From* Sugarbaker DJ, Bueno R, Colson YL, et al, editors. Adult Chest Surgery. 2nd edition. New York: The McGraw-Hill Company; 2015; with permission.)

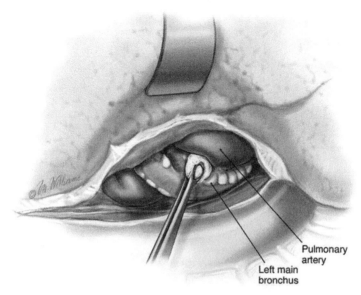

Pulmonary
artery

Left main
bronchus

Fig. 4. The pulmonary artery is dissected away from the bronchus posteriorly. (*From* Sugar-baker DJ, Bueno R, Colson YL, et al, editors. Adult Chest Surgery. 2nd edition. New York: The McGraw-Hill Company; 2015; with permission.)

attention not to injure the recurrent nerve or opening the pericardium to identify a very short left main pulmonary artery within the pericardium. When entering the pericardium to access the pulmonary artery, it is essential to test clamp the artery before it is divided because the anatomy may be distorted by the malignancy, which can lead to inadvertent division of the main pulmonary artery and disastrous consequences.

The left pulmonary artery may either be divided with a vascular stapler (**Fig. 5**)[43] or it may be occluded with a proximal and distal vascular clamps and manually cut. The pulmonary artery stump is sutured with a double layer of 5-0 Prolene.[44] In some cases, a combination of these techniques may be required.

Next the pulmonary veins are identified and divided. If the tumor invades the pericardium, or if the pericardium has been opened to gain arterial control, the veins can be controlled and divided by extending the pericardial opening inferiorly, just posterior to the phrenic nerve. The pulmonary veins form a single branch as they enter the left atrium and can be divided at this level with any of the techniques described for the artery (**Fig. 6**). When dividing the veins outside the pericardium, the superior and inferior veins must be identified separately. The inferior vein begins at the superior edge of the inferior pulmonary ligament, and the superior vein is the most anterior structure of the hilum. These veins can be divided with vascular stapler loads or controlled with vascular clamps and oversewn with 4-0 or 5-0 Prolene.

Attention should be paid to delicately dissect the bronchus and maintain its vascular supply to decrease the chances of bronchial stump leak with its attendant dangers. The bronchus is usually the last structure divided. The lung is grasped and used to deliver the bronchus into the chest, with the goal of dividing the left main bronchus just distal to the carina, while leaving sufficient length to avoid tension on the closure. This maneuver can be facilitated by dissection of the subcarinal lymph node packet. Next, the anesthesiologist is asked to hold ventilation and to back out the bronchial

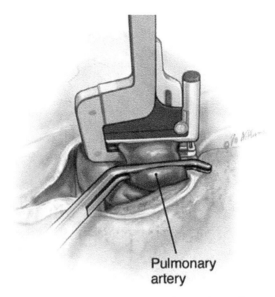

Pulmonary
artery

Fig. 5. The pulmonary artery is divided with a vascular stapler and a vascular clamp. (*From* Sugarbaker DJ, Bueno R, Colson YL, et al, editors. Adult Chest Surgery. 2nd edition. New York: The McGraw-Hill Company; 2015; with permission.)

blocker. The bronchial clamp or bronchial stapler is positioned across the bronchus to close it in an anterior-to-posterior fashion. If a stapler is used, the heavy load (green) or 4.8-mm stapler is chosen (**Fig. 7**). The anesthesiologist is then asked to ventilate the right lung to confirm correct positioning of the stapler. Once that is done and positioning of the stapler is indeed confirmed, ventilation is held again and the bronchus is closed and divided with the stapler.[45] The bronchus must be tested to

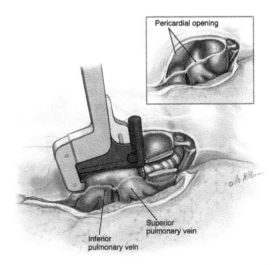

Pericardial opening

Superior
pulmonary vein

Inferior
pulmonary vein

Fig. 6. The pulmonary veins form a single branch as they enter the left atrium and are divided at this level when favorable anatomy is present. (*From* Sugarbaker DJ, Bueno R, Colson YL, et al, editors. Adult Chest Surgery. 2nd edition. New York: The McGraw-Hill Company; 2015; with permission.)

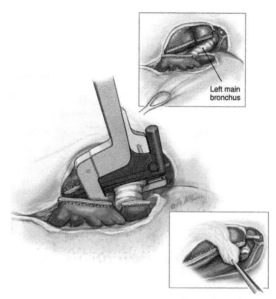

Fig. 7. The bronchus is usually the last structure divided with the goal of dividing the left main bronchus just distal to the carina. The bronchial clamp or bronchial stapler is positioned across the bronchus in an anterior-to-posterior fashion. If no leak is seen, the bronchus is covered with vascularized tissue. (*From* Sugarbaker DJ, Bueno R, Colson YL, et al, editors. Adult Chest Surgery. 2nd edition. New York: The McGraw-Hill Company; 2015; with permission.)

30 cm H_2O. If no leak is seen, the bronchus is covered with vascularized tissue. Whether an omental flap, a pericardial fat pad, a vascularized pericardium, or an intercostal muscle is used, it should be sutured either to the bronchus itself or to the tissues around the bronchus[46–49] (**Fig. 8**).

Right Pneumonectomy

Patients undergoing right pneumonectomy are more likely to die from this procedure than left pneumonectomy patients, typically owing to the complications of recovering from surgery rather than the surgery itself.[50,51] Consequently, for right pneumonectomy, postoperative management is crucial. As on the left side, a muscle-sparing posterolateral thoracotomy skin incision is made. The pleural space is approached via the fifth intercostal space and the chest cavity, chest wall, and lung are inspected for disease spread (see **Fig. 1**). The pleura around the hilum is divided and the inferior pulmonary ligament is taken down. For lesions in the hilum, dividing the azygos vein and harvesting the right paratracheal nodes first gives better exposure to the proximal pulmonary artery and proximal right mainstem bronchus (see **Fig. 8**). A patient who has had previous chemoradiation therapy or who has a history of granulomatous disease in the mediastinal lymph nodes often will have dense scarring between the posterior arterial plane and the anterior plane of the bronchus that will be encountered while dissecting the artery away from the bronchus and vein. Proximal control of the artery is needed when the surgeon encounters this situation.

Several maneuvers permit proximal control of the right main pulmonary artery; the simplest method is to divide the azygos vein and perform a right paratracheal node dissection. The proximal pulmonary artery can be approached by opening the

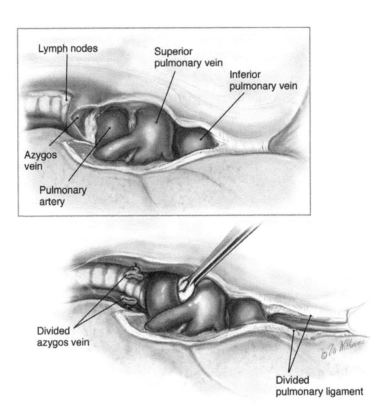

Fig. 8. For right-sided lesions in the hilum, dividing the azygos vein and harvesting the right paratracheal nodes first gives better exposure to the pulmonary artery and right mainstem bronchus. (*From* Sugarbaker DJ, Bueno R, Colson YL, et al, editors. Adult Chest Surgery. 2nd edition. New York: The McGraw-Hill Company; 2015; with permission.)

pericardium. Alternatively, the pulmonary artery can be identified medial to the superior vena cava, because the right main pulmonary artery is very long. The right pulmonary artery can be divided just after it crosses the aorta and the artery is then delivered back to the right hemithorax underneath the superior vena cava (**Fig. 9**). Notably, this approach markedly diminishes the chance of hemorrhage.

PERICARDIAL RESECTION AND RECONSTRUCTION

Pericardial reconstruction has been deemed necessary after pericardial resection during pneumonectomy, especially on the right side to prevent cardiac herniation.[52,53] However, owing to our experience of having patients arrest even after left sided pericardial resection, we believe the determining factor is the extent of resection rather than the side. The only goal of reconstruction is to repair the pericardial defect in a manner that would prevent herniation. Limited resections (<2 cm) may not require reconstruction to prevent herniation. Yet, reconstruction may be helpful in preventing tachyarrhythmias and in avoiding cardiac irritation. Most surgeons use a nonabsorbable material like Gore-Tex (W.L. Gore and Associates, Flagstaff, AZ) mesh to reconstruct the pericardium, whereas others fill the defect with some of the vascularized tissue flap used to buttress the bronchus. A Gore-Tex patch should be sewn into place

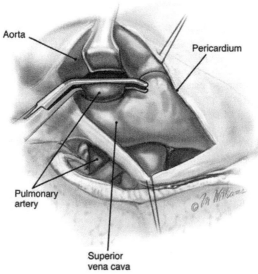

Fig. 9. The pulmonary artery is identified medial to the superior vena cava and divided just after its bifurcation and then delivered back to the right hemithorax underneath the superior vena cava. (*From* Sugarbaker DJ, Bueno R, Colson YL, et al, editors. Adult Chest Surgery. 2nd edition. New York: The McGraw-Hill Company; 2015; with permission.)

with interrupted sutures approximately 1 cm or more apart because the goal is to fix the patch in place and not to make it watertight (**Fig. 10**). This would avoid:

1. A state of positional pericardial constriction once the patient resumes upright position; and
2. Positional tension and narrowing of the superior vena cava as the patient changes positions.

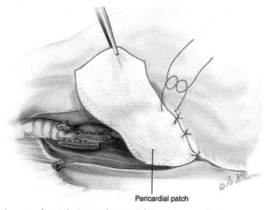

Pericardial patch

Fig. 10. The patch is sewn loosely into place with interrupted sutures approximately 1 cm or more apart. The desire is to fix the patch in place and not to make it watertight. (*From* Sugarbaker DJ, Bueno R, Colson YL, et al, editors. Adult Chest Surgery. 2nd edition. New York: The McGraw-Hill Company; 2015; with permission.)

PERIOPERATIVE MANAGEMENT

Postoperative management of the postpneumonectomy patient is beyond the scope of this article; however, some important points are worth mentioning. After pneumonectomy, and before leaving the operative theater, we place a 14-F red rubber catheter into the hemithorax and drain 500 to 1000 mL of air/fluid from the chest.[54] This helps to maintain a centered position of the mediastinum and allows for proper expansion of the contralateral lung. Serial chest radiographic monitoring and repeated drainage or insufflation of air is used to maintain proper positioning of the mediastinum in the first days after surgery.

A multidisciplinary team is essential to optimizing patient recovery in the perioperative period. Early mobilization after pneumonectomy has the known benefit of decreasing the risk of postoperative deep vein thrombosis, but also has the added benefit of contributing to effective pulmonary toilet and facilitating a shorter length of stay. Early extubation in the operating or recovery room is helpful at avoiding barotrauma to the staple line.

POSTOPERATIVE COMPLICATIONS

Pneumonectomy is a difficult and technically demanding operation associated with a high rate of perioperative morbidity.[15,25,55,56] Over time, perioperative mortality from pneumonectomy has decreased to 3% to 10% at select institutions.[57,58] This decrease is mainly attributed to increased awareness to the common postoperative complications and to improvement in the treatment provided these conditions. Good outcomes depend on a multidisciplinary team approach, awareness of the early signs of complications, and careful patient selection.

Careful preoperative patient evaluation will help to mitigate most of commonly encountered postoperative complications. Known risk factors for major postoperative complications include[26]:

- Age greater than 70 years
- High American Society of Anesthesiologists physical status
- Chronic obstructive pulmonary disease
- Coronary artery disease

The most common complications experienced after pneumonectomy are atrial fibrillation and vocal cord paralysis.[26,55,57]

Cardiac Complications

Atrial fibrillation

Atrial fibrillation has been reported to occur in up to 25% of postpneumonectomy patients and may manifest at any point during the postoperative hospital course.[59,60] Risk factors contributing to atrial fibrillation include large volume shifts intraoperatively and postoperatively, age greater than 65 years, pericardial resection with or without reconstruction, and right-sided pneumonectomies.[59] In patients with strong risk factors for developing postoperative atrial fibrillation the American Association for Thoracic Surgery recommends continuing beta-blocking agents if previously taking them, magnesium supplementation, diltiazem in patients with no known heart disease, or amiodarone in patients with some history of heart disease.[61] If postoperative atrial fibrillation should occur, treatment begins with optimizing fluid balance and maintaining a normal electrolyte profile. Hemodynamically unstable patients should be electrically cardioverted immediately, whereas hemodynamically stable patients can be treated with intravenous beta-blocking agents or calcium channel blockers to achieve a heart rate of less than 100 bpm.[61] A special mention should be made to anticoagulation of medically refractory atrial fibrillation after pneumonectomy. Because a postpneumonectomy patient can bleed almost their entire blood volume into the empty pleural space, any small bleeding vessel may lead to devastating consequences. Thus, consideration should be made to electrically cardiovert the patient in a timely manner. Notably, intracardiac thrombus formation should be ruled out before cardioversion.

Tamponade
Patients with symptoms of cardiac tamponade usually present with hypotension and increased filling pressures. This can be owing to a persistent pericardial effusion and/or a constrictive pericardial patch. A transesophageal echocardiogram can assess whether a constrictive effusion is present or whether the patch is too tight. Effusions are treated with either a pericardial window or a percutaneous drain.

Patch dysfunction
Constrictive patches require immediate reexploration and revision of the patch ensuring that there is a balance between the tension holding the patch in place and the laxity preventing restriction.[57]

Cardiac herniation
Cardiac herniation after pneumonectomy is rare. Causes include a loose patch, not using a patch after pericardial resection, sudden changes in intrathoracic pressure, chest tubes on suction, or sudden high peak airway pressures during mechanical ventilation.[55,62] An emergent thoracotomy is indicated should cardiac herniation occur. Once the patient is resuscitated, a return trip to the operating room should take place to wash out the chest and correct the underlying cause of the herniation. Special attention is warranted to make sure the pericardial patch is sewn to remaining pericardial tissue and not to weak tissue surrounding the pericardium.

Pulmonary Complications

Acute respiratory distress syndrome
Acute respiratory distress syndrome (ARDS) is a potentially fatal respiratory condition that presents with hypoxemia and stiff lungs.[63] It begins with alveolar capillary damage leading to increased endothelial permeability that results in the accumulation of protein rich fluid and neutrophils in the interstitium (fibroproliferative phase).[63,64] Recently, the European Society of Intensive Care Medicine, the American Thoracic Society and the Society of Critical Care Medicine revised the definition of ARDS, known as the Berlin definition. The revised definition states that[65]:

1. Symptoms must begin within 1 week of known insult or change in respiratory status
2. Bilateral opacities involving at least 3 quadrants, not fully explained by pleural effusions, atelectasis and nodules seen on chest radiography
3. Echocardiography or other objective test to rule out heart failure

The revised definition also clearly separates ARDS into mild, moderate, and severe according to the pulmonary arterial oxygen tension/fraction of inspired oxygen ratio while mechanically ventilated with a positive end-expiratory pressure of ≥ 5 cm H_2O.

ARDS occurs in 2% to 3% of postpneumonectomy patients with a distressing mortality rate of 50% to 70%.[56,66–69] Current treatment strategies for ARDS are supportive and include lung protective ventilation, diuresis, fluid restriction, and prone positioning.[63,70,71] The high mortality associated with ARDS highlights the importance of minimizing intraoperative and postoperative volume administration, and of perusing aggressive postoperative diuresis.

Empyema

Postpneumonectomy empyema occurs in 2% to 12% of standard postpneumonectomy patients and is usually associated with a bronchopleural fistula (BPF; addressed elsewhere in this article).[72] Known risk factors include advanced age, postoperative pneumonia, diabetes, steroids, induction chemoradiation, and malnutrition.[72] Treatment of postpneumonectomy empyema is time dependent. Early presentations (within the 1 month of pneumonectomy) can be managed safely with thoracoscopy, washout, debridement, and chest tube drainage of the hemithorax followed by postoperative antibiotic irrigation into the pneumonectomy space.[73] Patients who present months to years after pneumonectomy are treated with an open thoracostomy, long-term intravenous antibiotics, and eventual coverage using a pedicled muscle flap.

Bronchopleural fistula

BPFs are characterized by a direct communication between the trachea and the pneumonectomy space, with large fistulas leading to life threatening respiratory distress and sepsis. They occur in 1.7% to 11% of postpneumonectomy patients and mortality can be up to 40%.[46–49,74,75] BPFs share many of the same risk factors as postpneumonectomy empyemas, except that earlier fistulas (within 1 week of surgery) are often associated with technical failure to close the stump, or extensive dissection of the stump leading to devascularization.

BPFs presenting in the first or second postoperative days often require early revision of the stump in the operating room. All BPFs and in particular those presenting more than 48 hours after the operation should be considered infected and require similar measures of action as postpneumonectomy empyema. We initially place a chest tube for immediate drainage, send cultures of the pleural fluid, and start broad-spectrum antibiotics. Next, we perform a thoracostomy with stump coverage to protect the remaining lung from exposure to the ongoing infection. At the same time, we do not hesitate to place a jejunostomy tube to aid in nutrition optimization if the patient is malnourished. Once the infection has resolved, the thoracotomy space is filled with a muscle flap; thoracoplasty has been used with some success by other groups.[76] Small BPFs may occasionally respond to therapy with sclerosing agents like ethanol or injection of a fibrin glue.[77,78] As mentioned, BPF is a very serious and dangerous complication of lung resection in general and pneumonectomy in particular. Thus, BPF requires special attention from the surgical team and medical staff and only by careful attention to details and by repeated assessment of the patient can this situation be addressed properly.

Postpneumonectomy syndrome

Postpneumonectomy syndrome is a rare, late complication of right-sided pneumonectomy caused by severe shifting of the mediastinum to the right years after resection. The trachea is deviated to the right, causing the left mainstem bronchus to become impinged between the spine and the pulmonary artery. Tracheobronchomalacia occurs owing to the constant stretch and compression of the airway. Patients present with dyspnea, decreased exercise tolerance, and inspiratory stridor years after their pneumonectomy.[79] Treatment consists of filling the right hemithorax with an inert material (ie, acrylic balls) or using tissue expanders.[79,80]

QUALITY OF LIFE

One of the first questions patients have after being diagnosed with lung cancer is what of quality of life they will have. Pneumonectomy has been portrayed as the procedure of last resort when all hope is lost. Patients have little to no expectation of any quality of life and resign themselves to mental confinement by their disease. However, it is the duty of the surgeon to have an upfront and honest conversation with patients before surgery. Previous experience with pneumonectomy resulting in a poor quality of life was derived from inferior techniques and poor patient selection.[81] Multidisciplinary teams, improved surgical techniques, and more accurate clinical staging have selected out patients who would benefit most from a pneumonectomy. Cerfolio and colleagues[82] have recently looked at the quality of life experienced by patients after pneumonectomy and found that patients who have a good quality of life before surgery are likely to have a good quality of life after surgery. Age greater than 70 years and low preoperative quality of life were associated with poorer quality scores.[83] This is a significant change in the thought paradigm concerning pneumonectomy, where now the preoperative status of the patient drives the overall quality of life rather than burden of the surgery. As long as the surgeon performs a technically sound operation, there is no reason postpneumonectomy patients cannot go on to experience a good quality of life.

REFERENCES

1. Islami F, Tore LA, Jemal A. Global trends of lung cancer mortality and smoking prevalence. Transl Lung Cancer Res 2015;4(4):327–38.
2. Ettinger DS, Akerley W, Bepler G, et al. Non-small cell lung cancer. J Natl Compr Canc Netw 2010;8:740–801.
3. Detterbeck F, Postmus PE, Tanoue L. The stage classification of lung cancer. Chest 2013;143(Suppl 5):e191S–210S.
4. Jett J, Schild SE, Kesler K, et al. Treatment of small cell lung cancer. Chest 2013; 143(Suppl 5):e400S–19S.
5. Oser M, Niederst MJ, Sequist L, et al. Transformation from non-small-cell lung cancer to small-cell lung cancer: molecular drivers and cells of origin. Lancet Oncol 2015;16:e165–72.
6. Sugarbaker DJ, DaSilva MC. Diagnostic workup of lung cancer. Surg Oncol Clin 2011;20(4):667–79.
7. Ettinger D, Wood DE, Akerley W, et al. Non-small cell lung cancer: NCCN Guidelines. J Natl Compr Canc Netw 2015. Version 7. Available at: NCCN.org.
8. Howington J, Blum MG, Chang A, et al. Treatment of stage I and II non-small cell lung cancer: diagnosis and management of lung cancer, 3rd ed: American College of Chest Physicians evidence-based clinical practice guidelines. Chest 2013; 143(Suppl 5):e278S–313S.
9. Ramnath N, Dilling TJ, Harris L, et al. Treatment of Stage III Non-small Cell Lung Cancer: diagnosis and management of lung cancer, 3rd ed: American College of Chest Physicians evidence-based clinical practice guidelines. Chest 2013; 143(Suppl 5):e314S–40S.
10. Socinski M, Evans T, Gettinger S, et al. Treatment of Stage IV Non-small Cell Lung Cancer: Diagnosis and management of lung cancer, 3rd ed: American College of Chest Physicians evidence-based clinical practice guidelines. Chest 2013; 143(Suppl 5):e341S–68S.
11. Mery C, Pappas AN, Burt B, et al. Diameter of non-small cell lung cancer correlates with long-term survival: implications for T stage. Chest 2005;128: 3255–60.
12. Bordoni R. Consensus conference: multimodality management of early- and intermediate-stage non-small cell lung cancer. Oncologist 2008;13:945–53.

13. Samson P, Patel A, Crabtree T, et al. Multidisciplinary treatment for stage IIIA non-small cell lung cancer: does institution type matter? Ann Thorac Surg 2015; 100(5):1773–9.
14. Toyokawa G, Takenoyama M, Ichinose Y. Multimodality treatment with surgery for locally advanced non–small-cell lung cancer with N2 disease: a review article. Clin Lung Cancer 2015;16(1):6–14.
15. Wolf A, Daniel J, Sugarbaker D. Surgical techniques for multimodality treatment of malignant pleural mesothelioma: extrapleural pneumonectomy and pleurectomy/decortication. Semin Thorac Cardiovasc Surg 2009;21:132–48.
16. Yalman D. Neoadjuvant radiotherapy/chemoradiotherapy in locally advanced non-small cell lung cancer. Balkan Med J 2015;32(1):1–7.
17. Bott M, Patel AP, Crabtree T, et al. role for surgical resection in the multidisciplinary treatment of stage IIIB non–small cell lung cancer. Ann Thorac Surg 2015;99:1921–8.
18. Allen A, Mentzer SJ, Yeap B, et al. Pneumonectomy after chemoradiation. Cancer 2008;112:1106–13.
19. Tanaka S, Aoki M, Ishikawa H, et al. Pneumonectomy for node-positive non-small cell lung cancer: can it be a treatment option for N2 disease? Gen Thorac Cardiovasc Surg 2014;62:370–5.
20. Xu YP, Li B, Xu XL, et al. Is there a survival benefit in patients with stage IIIA (N2) non-small cell lung cancer receiving neoadjuvant chemotherapy and/or radiotherapy prior to surgical resection: a systematic review and meta-analysis. Medicine (Baltimore) 2015;94(23):e879.
21. Jaklitsch M, Herndon JE 2nd, Decamp M Jr, et al. Nodal downstaging predicts survival following induction chemotherapy for stage IIIA (N2) non-small cell lung cancer in CALGB Protocol #8935. J Surg Oncol 2006;94:599–606.
22. Gorenstein LA, Sonett JR. The surgical management of stage I and stage II lung cancer. Surg Oncol Clin N Am 2011;20(4):701–20.
23. Caglar H, Baldini EH, Othus M, et al. Outcomes of patients with stage III nonsmall cell lung cancer treated with chemotherapy and radiation with and without surgery. Cancer 2009;115:4156–66.
24. Elias A, Kumar P, Herndon J III, et al. Radiotherapy versus chemotherapy plus radiotherapy in surgically treated IIIA N2 non-small-cell lung cancer. Clin Lung Cancer 2002;4(2):95–103.
25. Al-Shahrabani F, Vallböhmer D, Angenendt S, et al. Surgical strategies in the therapy of non-small cell lung cancer. World J Clin Oncol 2014;5(4):595–603.
26. Alloubi I, Jougon J, Delcambre F, et al. Early complications after pneumonectomy: retrospective study of 168 patients. Interact Cardiovasc Thorac Surg 2010;11: 162–5.
27. Marret E, Miled F, Bazelly B, et al. Risk and protective factors for major complications after pneumonectomy for lung cancer. Interact Cardiovasc Thorac Surg 2010;10:936–9.
28. Brunelli A, Kim AW, Berger KI, et al. Physiologic evaluation of the patient with lung cancer being considered for resectional surgery: diagnosis and management of lung cancer, 3rd ed: American College of Chest Physicians evidence-based clinical practice guidelines. Chest 2013;143(Suppl 5):e166S–90S.
29. Choi H, Mazzone P. Preoperative evaluation of the patient with lung cancer being considered for lung resection. Curr Opin Anaesthesiol 2015;28(1):18–25.
30. Spyratos D, Zarogoulidis P, Porpodis K, et al. Preoperative evaluation for lung cancer resection. J Thorac Dis 2014;6(Suppl 1):S162–6.

31. Pillai R, Ramalingam SS. Advances in the diagnosis and treatment of non–small cell lung cancer. Mol Cancer Ther 2014;13(3):557–64.
32. Figueiredo VR, Jacomelli M, Rodrigues AJ, et al. Current status and clinical applicability of endobronchial ultrasound-guided transbronchial needle aspiration. J Bras Pneumol 2013;39(2):226–37 [in Portuguese].
33. Ge X, Guan W, Han F, et al. Comparison of endobronchial ultrasound-guided fine needle aspiration and video-assisted mediastinoscopy for mediastinal staging of lung cancer. Lung 2015;193(5):757–66.
34. Wahidi MM, Herth F, Yasufuku K, et al. Technical aspects of endobronchial ultrasound guided transbronchial needle aspiration: CHEST Guideline and Expert Panel Report. Chest 2015. [Epub ahead of print].
35. Riquet M, Mordant P, Pricopi C, et al. A review of 250 ten-year survivors after pneumonectomy for non-small-cell lung cancer. Eur J Cardiothorac Surg 2014; 45(5):876–81.
36. Roberts JR, Blum MG, Arildsen R, et al. Prospective comparison of radiologic, thoracoscopic, and pathologic staging in patients with early non-small cell lung cancer. Ann Thorac Surg 1999;68(4):1154–8.
37. Ferguson M, Watson S, Johnson E, et al. Predicted postoperative lung function is associated with all-cause long-term mortality after major lung resection for cancer. Eur J Cardiothorac Surg 2014;45:600–4.
38. Wang JS. Relationship of carbon monoxide pulmonary diffusing capacity to postoperative cardiopulmonary complications in patients undergoing pneumonectomy. Kaohsiung J Med Sci 2003;19:437–46.
39. Chang M, Mentzer SJ, Colson Y, et al. Factors predicting poor survival after resection of stage IA non–small cell lung cancer. J Thorac Cardiovasc Surg 2007;134:850–6.
40. Boysen PG, Harris JO, Block AJ, et al. Prospective evaluation for pneumonectomy using perfusion scanning: follow-up beyond one year. Chest 1981;80(2):163–6.
41. Win T, Tasker AD, Groves AM, et al. Ventilation-perfusion scintigraphy to predict postoperative pulmonary function in lung cancer patients undergoing pneumonectomy. AJR Am J Roentgenol 2006;187(5):1260–5.
42. Zhu X, Zhao M, Liu C, et al. Prediction of the postoperative pulmonary function in lung cancer patients with borderline function using ventilation-perfusion scintigraphy. Nucl Med Commun 2012;33(3):283–7.
43. Hendriks J, Lauwers P, Van Schil P. Extrapericardial pneumonectomy. Multimed Man Cardiothorac Surg 2005;2005(628). mmcts.2004.000083.
44. Ma Q, Liu D, Guo Y, et al. Surgical techniques and results of the pulmonary artery reconstruction for patients with central non-small cell lung cancer. J Cardiothorac Surg 2013;8:219.
45. Zakkar M, Kanagasabay R, Hunt I. No evidence that manual closure of the bronchial stump has a lower failure rate than mechanical stapler closure following anatomical lung resection. Interact Cardiovasc Thorac Surg 2014;18(4):488–93.
46. Lindner M, Hapfelmeier A, Morresi-Hauf A, et al. Bronchial stump coverage and postpneumonectomy bronchopleural fistula. Asian Cardiovasc Thorac Ann 2010; 18(5):443–9.
47. Sachithanandan A, Badmanaban B. Post pneumonectomy bronchopleural fistula: is it the closure technique or the operative side that really matters? Interact Cardiovasc Thorac Surg 2011;12(4):562.
48. Taghavi S, Marta GM, Lang G, et al. Bronchial stump coverage with a pedicled pericardial flap: an effective method for prevention of postpneumonectomy bronchopleural fistula. Ann Thorac Surg 2005;79(1):284–8.

49. Ucvet A, Gursoy S, Sirzai S, et al. Bronchial closure methods and risks for bron-chopleural fistula in pulmonary resections: how a surgeon may choose the opti-mum method? Interact Cardiovasc Thorac Surg 2011;12(4):558–62.

50. Bernard A, Deschamps C, Allen MS, et al. Pneumonectomy for malignant dis-ease: factors affecting early morbidity and mortality. J Thorac Cardiovasc Surg 2001;121(6):1076–82.

51. Stolz AJ, Harustiak T, Simonek J, et al. Pneumonectomy for non-small cell lung cancer: predictors of early mortality and morbidity. Acta Chir Belg 2014;114(1):25–30.

52. Kawamukai K, Antonacci F, Di Saverio S, et al. Acute postoperative cardiac her-niation. Interact Cardiovasc Thorac Surg 2011;12(1):73–4.

53. Mehanna MJ, Israel GM, Katigbak M, et al. Cardiac herniation after right pneumo-nectomy: case report and review of the literature. J Thorac Imaging 2007;22(3):280–2.

54. Wolf A, Jacobson FL, Tilleman T, et al. Managing the pneumonectomy space after extrapleural pneumonectomy: postoperative intrathoracic pressure monitoring. Eur J Cardiothorac Surg 2010;37:770–5.

55. Sugarbaker D, Jaklitsch MT, Bueno R, et al. Prevention, early detection, and man-agement of complications after 328 consecutive extrapleural pneumonectomies. J Thorac Cardiovasc Surg 2004;128:138–46.

56. Dulu A, Pastores SM, Park B, et al. Prevalence and mortality of acute lung injury and ARDS after lung resection. Chest 2006;130(1):73–8.

57. Zellos L, Jaklitsch MT, Al-Mourgi M, et al. Complications of extrapleural pneumo-nectomy. Semin Thorac Cardiovasc Surg 2007;19:355–9.

58. Krasna MJ, Gamliel Z, BurrowsW, et al. Pneumonectomy for lung cancer after preoperative concurrent chemotherapy and high-dose radiation. Ann Thorac Surg 2010;89:200–6.

59. AJCC. Lung. In: Edge SB, Byrd DR, Compton CC, et al, editors. AJCC cancer staging manual. 7th edition. New York: Springer; 2010. p. 253–70.

60. Harpole DH, Liptay MJ, DeCamp MM Jr, et al. Prospective analysis of pneumo-nectomy: risk factors for major morbidity and cardiac dysrhythmias. Ann Thorac Surg 1996;61(3):977–82.

61. Frendl G, Sodickson AC, Chung MK, et al. 2014 AATS guidelines for the preven-tion and management of perioperative atrial fibrillation and flutter for thoracic sur-gical procedures. Executive summary. J Thorac Cardiovasc Surg 2014;148(3):772–91.

62. Harpole DH Jr, DeCamp MM Jr, Daley J, et al. Prognostic models of thirty-day mortality and morbidity after major pulmonary resection. J Thorac Cardiovasc Surg 1999;117(5):969–79.

63. Fanelli V, Vlachou A, Ghannadian S, et al. Acute respiratory distress syndrome: new definition, current and future therapeutic options. J Thorac Dis 2013;5(3):326–34.

64. Matthay MA, Ware LB, Zimmerman GA. The acute respiratory distress syndrome. J Clin Invest 2012;122(8):2731–40.

65. ARDS Definition Task Force, Ranieri VM, Rubenfeld GD, et al. Acute respiratory distress syndrome: the Berlin definition. JAMA 2012;307:2526–33.

66. Parquin F, Marchal M, Mehiri S, et al. Post-pneumonectomy pulmonary edema: analysis and risk factors. Eur J Cardiothorac Surg 1996;10(11):929–32 [discus-sion: 933].

67. Kutlu CA, Williams EA, Evans TW, et al. Acute lung injury and acute respiratory distress syndrome after pulmonary resection. Ann Thorac Surg 2000;69(2): 376–80.
68. Tang SS, Redmond K, Griffiths M, et al. The mortality from acute respiratory distress syndrome after pulmonary resection is reducing: a 10-year single institutional experience. Eur J Cardiothorac Surg 2008;34(4):898–902.
69. Pricopi C, Mordant P, Rivera C. Postoperative morbidity and mortality after pneumonectomy: a 30-year experience of 2064 consecutive patients. Interact Cardiovasc Thorac Surg 2015;20(3):316–21.
70. Ventilation with lower tidal volumes as compared with traditional tidal volumes for acute lung injury and the acute respiratory distress syndrome. The Acute Respiratory Distress Syndrome Network. N Engl J Med 2000;342(18):1301–8.
71. Guerin C, Reignier J, Richard JC, et al. Prone positioning in severe acute respiratory distress syndrome. N Engl J Med 2013;368(23):2159–68.
72. Van Schil PE, Hendriks JM, Lauwers P. Focus on treatment complications and optimal management surgery. Transl Lung Cancer Res 2014;3(3):181–6.
73. Gossot D, Stern JB, Galetta D, et al. Thoracoscopic management of postpneumonectomy empyema. Ann Thorac Surg 2004;78(1):273–6.
74. Groth SS, Burt BM, Sugarbaker DJ. Management of complications after pneumonectomy. Thorac Surg Clin 2015;25(3):335–48.
75. Jichen QV, Chen G, Jiang G, et al. Risk factor comparison and clinical analysis of early and late bronchopleural fistula after non-small cell lung cancer surgery. Ann Thorac Surg 2009;88(5):1589–93.
76. Stefani A, Jouni R, Alifano M, et al. Thoracoplasty in the current practice of thoracic surgery: a single-institution 10-year experience. Ann Thorac Surg 2011;91(1): 263–8.
77. Takaoka K, Inoue S, Ohira S. Central bronchopleural fistulas closed by bronchoscopic injection of absolute ethanol. Chest 2002;122(1):374–8.
78. Glover W, Chavis TV, Daniel TM, et al. Fibrin glue application through the flexible fiberoptic bronchoscope: closure of bronchopleural fistulas. J Thorac Cardiovasc Surg 1987;93(3):470–2.
79. Jansen JP, Brutel de la Riviere A, Alting MP, et al. Postpneumonectomy syndrome in adulthood. Surgical correction using an expandable prosthesis. Chest 1992; 101(4):1167–70.
80. Haithcock BE, Feins RH. Complications of pulmonary resection. In: Shields TW, LoCicero J III, Reed CE, et al, editors. General thoracic surgery. 7th edition. Philadelphia: Lippincott Williams & Wilkins; 2009. p. 551–9.
81. Leo F, Scanagatta P, Vannucci F, et al. Impaired quality of life after pneumonectomy: who is at risk? J Thorac Cardiovasc Surg 2010;139(1):49–52.
82. Cerfolio RJ, Bryant AS. Quality of life after pulmonary resections. Thorac Surg Clin 2013;23(3):437–42.
83. Bryant AS, Cerfolio RJ, Minnich DJ. Survival and quality of life at least 1 year after pneumonectomy. J Thorac Cardiovasc Surg 2012;144(5):1139–43.

Stereotactic Body Radiotherapy and Ablative Therapies for Lung Cancer

Ghulam Abbas, MD, MHCM, FACS[a],*, Adnan Danish, MD[b],
Mark J. Krasna, MD[c]

KEYWORDS

- Stereotactic body radiation therapy (SBRT) • Radiofrequency ablation
- Microwave ablation • Ablative therapies for lung cancer
- Stereotactic ablative therapy (SABR)

KEY POINTS

- The treatment paradigm for early stage lung cancer and oligometastatic disease to the lung is rapidly changing.
- Ablative therapies, especially SABR, are challenging the surgical gold standard and have the potential to be the standard for operable patients with early stage lung cancer who are high risk for morbidities.
- Microwave ablation is another promising novel ablative modality that in the near future would also be available for transbronchial ablation of small lung tumors, especially more central tumors.
- The outcome results of the ablative therapies should be compared with anatomic minimally invasive segmentectomy or lobectomy with lymph node dissection rather than historical surgical data.

Lung cancer remains the leading cause of cancer-related death in men and women in United States.[1] Surgical resection offers the best chance of cure in early stage disease. Surgical resection is also beneficial in a select group of patients with limited pulmonary metastases. Unfortunately, most patients with lung cancer present with advanced-stage disease and are not surgically curable. Among the patients with early stage lung cancer, more than 20% cannot tolerate surgery because of comorbid conditions.[2] Similarly, some patients with limited pulmonary metastases, who would benefit from metasectomy, are deemed high-risk secondary to poor cardiopulmonary reserves.

Disclosure Statement: The authors have nothing to disclose.
[a] Minimally Invasive Thoracic Surgery, Meridian Health, 1 Riverview Plaza, Red Bank, NJ 07701, USA; [b] Radiation Oncology, Meridian Health, 1 Riverview Plaza, Red Bank, NJ 07701, USA; [c] Meridian Cancer Care, Jersey Shore University Medical Center, Ackerman South, Room 553, 1945 Route 33, Neptune, NJ 07753, USA
* Corresponding author. 1 Riverview Plaza, Red Bank, NJ 07733.
E-mail address: gabbas@meridianhealth.com

Surg Oncol Clin N Am 25 (2016) 553–566
http://dx.doi.org/10.1016/j.soc.2016.02.008
1055-3207/16/$ – see front matter © 2016 Elsevier Inc. All rights reserved.

External beam radiation therapy may be offered as an alternate to surgery in patients with limited-stage disease who are too high-risk for surgery. However, reported 5-year survival with this modality is only 10% to 30%.[3,4] The outcome data for stage I non–small cell cancer (NSCLC), treated with radiation therapy alone, from Duke University in 156 patients showed 2- and 5-year survival rates of 39% and 13%, respectively. In a study of 71 node-negative patients who received at least 60 Gy of radiotherapy, 3- and 5-year survivals were 19% and 12%, respectively.[4] Another concern with external beam radiation is radiation pneumonitis, which is a potentially life threatening complication in these severely impaired patients. Zierhut and colleagues,[5] in their study of 60 patients with NSCLC, reported an 8.3% incidence of radiation pneumonitis in patients treated with definitive radiotherapy. Several studies have reported a benefit to dose escalation with a dose-response relationship for local control and survival. When dose escalation is attempted using conventional treatment techniques, however, dose-limiting toxicity occurs. Increased doses of radiation result in increased toxicity and damage to surrounding pulmonary parenchyma, which limits safe dose escalation.[6,7] Dose-volume histogram data show a correlation between risk of pulmonary toxicity and indices of dose to lung parenchyma. The risk of toxicity increases as the area of irradiated adjacent normal lung increases.[8–10] Radiation fibrosis seems to depend on the volume of the lung that is radiated above a threshold of 20 Gy to 30 Gy and dose escalation is limited primarily by the risk of radiation pneumonitis.

Over the last two decades, ablative alternatives to resection or standard external beam radiation therapy have been introduced into clinical practice for the treatment of limited-stage lung cancer or limited pulmonary metastases. The most common modalities offered by many centers around the world are stereotactic body radiotherapy (SBRT), microwave ablation (MWA), radiofrequency ablation (RFA), cryotherapy, photodynamic therapy, and irreversible electrophoresis.

STEREOTACTIC BODY RADIOTHERAPY

SBRT, also known as stereotactic ablative therapy (SABR), holds the most potential for curative radiotherapy in patients with early stage lung tumors. Stereotactic targeting uses a variety of systems to decrease the effects of lung motion, which translate into target motion, and improve localization techniques by collection of precise measurements to account for tumor motion during treatment planning and delivery of each fraction. These systems allow dramatic reduction of treatment volume, facilitating hypofractionation with markedly increased daily doses and a significantly reduced overall treatment time and decreased irradiation of normal surrounding tissues with an associated reduction in toxicity. This is possible because radiation can be precisely contoured to the tumor with a very rapid fall-off of radiation in the surrounding lung parenchyma. Treatment is typically delivered in three to five fractions over a 1- to 2-week period, ranging on average from 10 Gy to 20 Gy per fraction. The resulting biologic effective dose (BED) of SBRT is typically in excess of 100 Gy, in contrast to a BED of 79.2 Gy with standard fractionation.[11,12]

Currently there are a variety of platforms available for SABR. Some of these systems, especially Acuray Cyberknife (Accuray, Sunnyvale, CA), need placement of gold fiducial for image-guided tumor location during treatment. These can either be placed percutaneously using computed tomography (CT) guidance or transbronchially using navigational bronchoscopy (Electromagnetic Navigation Bronchoscopy, Medtronic, Dublin, Ireland). CT-guided fiducial placement is done under local anesthesia and is complicated by pneumothorax in 13% to 47% of cases. Electromagnetic

Navigation Bronchoscopy system is used to place the fiducials around the tumor transbronchially. This technique is associated with less incidence of pneumothorax.

Clinical Results

In one of the earliest studies from Indiana University, Timmerman and colleagues[13] reported the outcome of a phase I dose escalation toxicity study. In this trial 47 medically inoperable patients with T1 and T2 NSCLC were treated with SBRT. Patients were treated with three fractions administered over a 2-week period using a frame-based radiosurgery system. The doses started at 8 Gy per fraction and were escalated to 20 Gy. At a median follow-up of 15.2 months, no late toxicity attributable to therapy was identified. Complete response was seen in 27% of patients and partial response was seen in 60%. With a 15-month follow-up, more than one-third (13 of 37) of patients showed progression of cancer. Among these 13 patients with cancer progression, six (6 of 13) showed local recurrence. These local recurrences were observed more commonly at lower radiation doses and occurred at a median of 13 months after treatment. A superior response rate of 87% with dose escalation was also noted. No patient treated with greater than 18 Gy per fraction showed progression during short-term follow-up.

A phase II trial from the same institution further evaluated efficacy and safety of SABR in this patient population.[14] Doses established in the phase I trial were used to treat 70 patients with stage I NSCLC. For the initial report, 2-year local control was 95%, with a median follow-up of 17.5 months, and overall survival (OS) was 56% at 2 years. Most of the deaths were related to comorbid illnesses seen in this inoperable population, rather than death associated with lung cancer; however, there were six treatment-related deaths. Severe toxicity (grades 3–5) was seen in a greater proportion of patients with "central" tumors, defined as tumors near the proximal bronchial tree (see section on toxicity). The report was later updated after a median follow-up of 50 months, showing 3-year local control and survival of 88% and 42%, respectively.

In the Radiation Therapy Oncology Group (RTOG) 0236 protocol, 55 patients with peripheral, less than 5 cm (T1-T2, N0) tumors were treated with three fractions of 18 Gy with total dose of 54 Gy.[15] Eleven patients had distant metastasis within 1 year of treatment and 22% had disseminated recurrence at the end of 3 years. Although the local control rates were high, the 3 years disease-free and OS rates were 48% and 56%, respectively.

At the American Society of Radiation Oncology's 56th annual meeting, Timmerman and colleagues[16] presented updated 5-year data from the RTOG 0236 trial. The updated results showed a local recurrence rate of 20%, caused primarily by intralobar recurrence. Additionally, 5-year locoregional and distant recurrence rates were 38% and 31%, respectively. The high incidence of recurrence is probably caused by less optimal staging and use of less than 100 BED doses during RTOG 0236 protocol.

The University of Pittsburgh radiation oncology and thoracic surgery groups have successfully proven a model in which patients for SABR are evaluated by the radiation oncologist and thoracic surgeon. In their early experience, they reported the results of 32 patients treated with CyberKnife stereotactic radiosurgery.[17] They subsequently analyzed 21 medically inoperable patients with stage I NSCLC that were treated with a median dose of 20 Gy in a single fraction using the Cyberknife system.[18] An initial response was observed in 12 patients (12 of 21; 57%), and disease was stable in five (5 of 21; 24%), progressed in three (3 of 21; 14%), and was not evaluable in one (one of 21; 5%). At a mean follow-up of 24 months, the estimated probability of survival at 1-year was 81% (confidence interval [CI], 0.73–0.90). The median survival was

26.4 months (95% CI, 19.6 [not reached]). Local progression occurred in nine patients (42%). The median time to local progression was 12.3 months. This led to the adoption of a more aggressive protocol where all peripheral tumors were treated with 60 Gy in three fractions and more central tumors were treated with 48 Gy in four fractions. Recently they published their outcomes using SABR for recurrent lung neoplasms in 100 patients.[19] The postprocedure 30-day mortality was 0%; median follow-up was 51 months. The median OS for the entire group was 23 months (95% CI, 19–41 months). The probability of 2- and 5-year OS was 49% (95% CI, 40%–60%) and 31% (95% CI, 23%–43%), respectively.

Multiple studies have shown that BED of 100 Gy or more leads to better outcomes with less local recurrence. Onishi and colleagues[20] reported on an amalgamation of multi-institutional data from Japan that included 257 patients (164 patients with stage IA disease and 93 with stage IB disease) with a median tumor size of 2.8 cm (range, 0.7–5.8 cm). The median follow-up period for the entire cohort was 38 months. The patients were divided into two groups based on the dose they received, 215 patients received 100 Gy BED and the other 42 patients received less than 100 Gy BED. The overall local control rate for the entire cohort was 86%. The group that received 100 Gy BED had a local control rate of 91.6%, whereas those who received a BED less than 100 Gy had a local control rate of only 57.1% ($P<.001$). The 3- and 5-year OS for the entire cohort was 56.8% and 47.2%, respectively. The 3-year OS rate in medically operable patients was 88.4% for BED greater than 100 Gy compared with 69.4% for less than 100 Gy. The 5-year OS for the BED 100 Gy cohort was 53.9%, compared with only 19.7% for less than 100 Gy ($P<.05$).

In another Japanese trial, Japan Clinical Oncology Group 0403, Nagata and colleagues[21] initially published the results inoperable patients in 2010,[22] in operable in 2012, and follow-up in 2015.[23] The aim of the study was to evaluate the safety and efficacy of SBRT in patients with histologically or cytologically proven NSCLC. Between July 2004 and November 2008, a total of 169 patients from 15 institutions were registered. One hundred inoperable and 64 operable patients (total 164) were eligible. Patient characteristics were 122 male and 47 female; median age, 78 years (range, 50–91 years); and 90 adenocarcinomas, 61 squamous cell carcinomas, and 18 others. Of the 100 inoperable patients, the 3-year OS was 59.9%. Grade 3 and 4 toxicities were observed in 10 and 2 patients, respectively. No grade 5 toxicity was observed. The 3-year OS for operable patients was better and was 76.5%. The progression-free survival was 54.5%. Grade 3 toxicities were observed in five patients. No grade 4 and 5 toxicities were observed.

RTOG protocol 0618[24] was a phase II trial using SBRT to treat early stage NSCLC in operable patients (deemed surgically resectable). Patients with biopsy-proven peripheral T1 to T3 tumors were treated with 18 Gy in three fractions delivered in 2 weeks. The study opened December 2007 and closed May 2010 after accruing a total of 33 patients. Of 26 evaluable patients, 23 had T1 and three had T2 tumors. Median age was 72 years. Four patients (16%) had SBRT-related grade 3 toxicity, whereas none had grade 4 to 5 adverse events. Median follow-up was 25 months. Two-year estimates of local failure, regional failure, and distant failure were 19.2%, 11.7%, and 15.4%, respectively. Two-year estimates of progression-free survival and OS are 65.4% and 84.4%, respectively.

The results of RTOG 0915 trial were recently published.[25] This was a randomized phase II study comparing two SBRT schedules for medically inoperable patients with stage I peripheral NSCLC. The aim of the study was to compare two SBRT schedules for medically inoperable early stage lung cancer to determine which produces the lowest rate of grade 3 and higher protocol-specified adverse events at 1 year. Patients with biopsy-proven peripheral T1 or T2 were randomized either to receive 34 Gy in one fraction (arm 1) or 48 Gy in four consecutive daily fractions (arm 2). Ninety-four patients were accrued between September 2009 and March 2011. The median follow-up time was 30.2 months. Of 84 analyzable patients, 39 were in arm 1 and 45 in arm 2. Four (10.3%) patients on arm 1 and six (13.3%) patients on arm 2 experienced adverse events. The 2-year OS and disease-free survival rate was 61.3% and 56.4% for arm 1 and 77.7% and 71% for arm 2. The short follow-up is the major limitation of this study because the adverse events, such as pneumonitis, rib fracture, and nerve injury, can happen beyond 1 year posttreatment. The survival seems to be better with multi-fraction rather than single fraction arm 2. Until further comparison is performed patients should be treated in three to five fractions.

COMPARING STEREOTACTIC ABLATIVE THERAPY WITH SURGERY

The encouraging results with good outcome in medically inoperable patients led to the enthusiasm of using SBRT for medically operable patients and also comparing this modality with surgical resection, which is the gold standard for the treatment of early stage lung cancer.

In an earlier retrospective comparison of 464 patients who underwent surgery and 76 who underwent SABR for clinical stage I NSCLC, local control at 3 years was improved with surgery for stage IA patients (96% vs 89%; $P = .04$) but no different for stage IB patients ($P = .89$).[26] Although no difference in disease-specific survival was seen, surgery was associated with improved OS ($P<.001$). In their updated T-stage matched analysis of patients treated with lobar resection (N = 260) or SBRT (N = 78), there was no significant difference in patterns of failure or cause-specific survival, whereas OS favored surgery.[27]

Multiple studies from the Netherlands have compared surgery with SABR. In a propensity score–matched analysis based on stage, age, gender, comorbidity score, lung function, and performance status, locoregional control rates were higher in patients receiving SABR (N = 64) than those receiving video-assisted thoracoscopic surgery (VATS) (N = 64) (86.9% vs 82.6%; $P = .04$), whereas there was no difference in distant recurrence rate or OS.[28] The less than desired outcome in the VATS group may be caused by the institution's early experience with VATS (adopted VATS in 2007) and less aggressive lymph node dissection with only 70% having more than five lymph nodes harvested. In an updated propensity score–matched analysis (N = 73 for each modality), survival was similar ($P = .089$) at 12 months (95% vs 94%) and 60 months (80% vs 53%) for patients undergoing surgery and SABR, with a trend toward improved survival with surgery at longer follow-up identified.[29] Another recent publication from the Netherlands evaluated the outcome of patients with stage I (T1 and T2) NSCLC treated with surgery (N = 143) or SABR (N = 197); survival was similar across modalities when controlling for prognostic covariables ($P = .73$). When examining recurrences, local and distant control were similar but locoregional recurrences occurred more following SABR ($P = .028$), suggesting a need to improve staging in SABR.[30]

In the United States, Surveillance, Epidemiology, and End Results (SEER) studies have also compared surgery with SABR. Among 10,923 patients aged greater than or equal to 66 years with stage I NSCLC treated from 2001 to 2007, most (59%) were treated with lobectomy, whereas only 1.1% were treated with SABR. SABR was associated with a lower risk of death at 6 months, whereas lobectomy had better long-term survival.[30] On propensity score–matched analysis, SABR and lobectomy had similar survivals. Similarly, a SEER study of 9093 patients with stage I NSCLC treated from 2003 to 2009 with lobectomy (79.3%), sublobar resection (16.5%), or SABR (4.2%) reported unadjusted 90-day mortality to be highest with lobectomy and lowest with SABR (4.0% vs 1.3%; $P = .008$). However, at 3 years, unadjusted mortality was lowest with surgery (25.0% vs 45.1%; $P<.001$), showing better long-term survival with surgery.[31]

Based on the highly promising outcome of SBRT in medically inoperable patients, three randomized trials comparing SBRT with lobectomy (ROSEL, STAR) or sublobar resection (American College of Surgery Oncology Group [ACOSOG] Z4099/RTOG 1021) have been started but all three studies closed very early because of poor accrual: less than 5% of the planned patients were enrolled.

STEREOTACTIC RADIOTHERAPY VS SURGERY AND RADIOSURGERY OR SURGERY FOR OPERABLE EARLY STAGE NON-SMALL CELL LUNG CANCER TRIALS

STARS (StereoTActic Radiotherapy vs. Surgery) is an international randomized phase III trial comparing CyberKnife SABR with surgical resection. ROSEL (Radiosurgery Or Surgery for operable Early stage non-small cell Lung cancer) is a randomized phase III trial by VU Medical Centre Amsterdam and the Dutch Lung Cancer Research Group comparing SABR with surgery.

In the STARS trial, patients with tumors smaller than 4 cm and operable clinical stage I NSCLC received either surgical resection and mediastinal lymph node dissection or SABR to 54 Gy in three fractions for peripheral tumors or 50 Gy in four fractions for central tumors.

In the ROSEL trial, patients with tumors less than 3 cm with operable clinical stage IA NSCLC received either surgical resection (lobectomy was preferred but limited resection was acceptable) or SABR to 54 Gy in three fractions for peripheral tumors or 60 Gy in five fractions for central tumors. Histologic confirmation of an NSCLC diagnosis was required in the STARS trial but not the ROSEL trial, although lesions had to be new or growing and radiographically consistent with NSCLC and avidity on PET/CT.

Although the STARS and ROSEL trials closed early because of poor accrual, a pooled analysis of the two trials was conducted by Chang and colleagues[32] with a primary outcome of OS. Fifty-eight patients were enrolled and randomized to SABR (N = 31) or surgery (N = 27, 5 VATS and 22 thoracotomy), with no differences in patient or tumor characteristics found between arms. OS was found to be significantly higher among patients randomized to SABR with 3-year survival of 95% versus 79% for surgical patients. This survival difference was significant in the STARS trial alone ($P = .0067$) but not the ROSEL trial ($P = .78$). At 3 years, there was no difference in local control (SABR 96% vs surgery 100%; $P = .44$), regional nodal control (90% vs 96%; $P = .32$), metastatic-free survival (97% vs 91%; $P = .42$), and recurrence-free survival (86% vs 80%; $P = .54$). These results should be interpreted with caution because the STARS trial only enrolled 36 of its intended 1030 patients and the ROSEL trial only enrolled 22 of its intended 960 patients. Also 5 of 27 patients had VATS and the rest had thoracotomy probably associated with higher morbidity and poorer outcome.

A SURGEON'S VIEW

Several well-designed prospective studies have clearly proven that SABR is safe and effective for medically inoperable and operable patients with NSCLC. However, the results of these studies should be interpreted with caution. The results of SABR outcomes are usually compared with the historical surgical outcomes rather than contemporary outcomes of minimally invasive surgery. In these series, preoperative staging was less accurate because of nonexistent modern imaging technology. Also morbidity and mortality was higher because minimally invasive surgery for lung cancer has only matured recently. In the United States almost half of the lung cancer resections are performed by surgeons who are not trained in thoracic oncology, leading to less optimal decision-making and oncologic resection. The less aggressive lymph node dissection may lead to higher recurrence and decreased survival.

Multiple studies have shown that 20% to 30% of stage I lung cancers are upgraded during surgery because of occult N1 or N2 disease.[33–35] These patients are at a disadvantage if treated with SABR because their nodal status is unknown and are at higher risk for recurrence without adjuvant systematic treatment.

A retrospective analysis using SEER data suggests SABR is superior to sublobar resection.[31] There are excellent outcome studies from Japan and the United States showing anatomic segmentectomy for stage 1A lung cancer has the same recurrence and survival rates as lobectomy with less morbidity, especially in older patients.[33] It is misleading to compare the well-organized prospective SABR data with historical surgical outcomes or SEER data.

Similarly, how recurrence is defined is different in SABR data versus surgical literature. SABR literature refers to local recurrence as recurrence at the primary tumor site. However, local failure in surgical series has generally included recurrence within the same lobe away from the primary site (regarded as distant failure in many SABR experiences), and may include recurrence within an ipsilateral nonprimary lobe, usually hilar lymph nodes.

Another factor that must be considered is how local failure is identified. After SABR, residual scarring may remain in the lung, and the challenge is differentiating this from viable tumor. Biopsy may be difficult, and so serial imaging provides the best estimation of potential recurrence. However, in a high-risk group of patients, death may occur from another cause, before growth is appreciated in a region of viable tumor, therefore underestimating the incidence of recurrent disease (ask affect overall but not recurrence-free survival).

Another concern is the selection of patients deemed medically inoperable or high-risk operable. An analysis comparing the patient populations from three cooperative group studies included patients from Z4032, a study of high-risk operable patients treated with sublobar resection; Z4033, a study of medically inoperable patients treated with RFA; and RTOG 0236, a study of medically inoperable patients treated with SABR.[36] The Z4032 and Z4033 studies had similar inclusion criteria, except that an ACOSOG-approved surgeon had to declare the patient medically inoperable to enter Z4033. The Z4033 patients were significantly older and had the worst predicted carbon monoxide diffusion capacity compared with the other groups. The best pulmonary function was reported in the RTOG 0236 patients showing challenges in comparing these different modalities for the treatment of early stage lung cancer.

Future Trials

The ACOSOG Z4099/RTOG 1021 randomized phase III trial of sublobar resection with or without brachytherapy versus SABR in high-risk patients with stage I NSCLC, the only other phase III randomized trial conducted to date other than the STARS and ROSEL trials, is unlikely to provide any significant additional insight in the debate of SABR versus surgery given that it closed early in 2013 because of lack of accrual and is without publication. However, additional insight from two upcoming randomized trials may be forthcoming. The VALOR trial (Veterans Affairs Lung cancer surgery Or stereotactic Radiotherapy) is scheduled to open in the United States within the year, and the SABRTooth trial (a multicenter pilot and feasibility study that will compare SABR and surgery for peripheral stage I NSCLC in patients thought to be at higher risk of surgical complications) is also planned to open in the United Kingdom.

Toxicity of Treatment

Although SABR is safe and usually without any short-term adverse effects, it may lead to significant delayed morbidity or even death. A study by Timmerman and colleagues[14] reported the outcome of 70 patients with T1 or T2 less than 7-cm tumors, treated with high-dose stereotactic radiosurgery. T1 tumors were treated with 60 Gy in three fractions and T2 tumors were treated with 66 Gy in three fractions. Fifty-eight of 70 patients had grade 1 to 2 toxicity consisting mostly of fatigue, musculoskeletal discomfort, and radiation pneumonitis, which was sometimes treated with oral corticosteroids. Most grade 1 to 2 toxicities occurred within 1 to 2 months of treatment and resolved by 3 to 4 months posttreatment. Eight patients had grade 3 to 4 toxicity as evidenced by decrease in pulmonary function tests, pneumonias, pleural effusions, apnea, and skin reactions. The time from treatment to toxicity for these more severe toxicities was a median of 7.6 months. Four of the six deaths were seen in patients with central or perihilar tumors. Central and perihilar tumors had an 11 times increased risk of toxicity. Size of the gross tumor volume was also a significant predictor of grade 3 to 5 toxicity. Tumors with gross tumor volumes greater than 10 mL had an eight times increased risk of high-grade toxicity versus smaller tumors. Survival was worse in patients with T2 tumors, worse in patients with cardiac comorbidities compared with pulmonary comorbidities, and worse in patients with a forced expiratory volume in 1 second less than 40%. The authors concluded that treatment with 60 Gy in three fractions to central tumors may be too toxic.

MICROWAVE ABLATION

MWA is a relatively recent development in the approach to tumor ablation. The mechanism of MWA is dielectric heating (frictional heating of water molecules in tissue). As microwave radiation interacts with water molecules, the polarity of these molecules changes resulting in heating and eventually leading to cell death.

MWA is slowly replacing RFA for thermal ablation of lung tumors. In comparison with RFA, MWA leads to enhanced thermocoagulation of tumor cells as a result of improved energy deposition in the lung, higher temperatures within the tumor in a shorter amount of time, and a larger ablative area. MWA may allow for improved treatment of central lesions compared with RFA because of minimal heat sink effect associated with surrounding vasculature. The most common complications of MWA are similar to those of RFA, including risk of pneumothorax, postprocedure pain, and hemoptysis.

Clinical experience with MWA for lung tumors is limited at this time. Feng and colleagues[37] reported on MWA of 28 tumors in 20 patients. A response of 50% ablation or more was noted in 13 (46.4%) nodules and a complete response in three (10.7%). No significant complications were noted. An ablate and resect study was performed by Simon and colleagues.[38] Patients undergoing elective lung resection underwent MWA before their resection. The mean tumor diameter was 3 cm (range, 2–5.5 cm) with an average tumor volume of 7.1 cm^3. The mean maximum ablation achieved was 4 cm (range, 3–5 cm), with an average tumor volume of 23.4 cm^3. Wolf and colleagues[39] reported their results of MWA in 82 lung tumors of 50 patients. At a mean follow-up of 10 months, 26% of the patients had residual disease at the ablation site and another 22% had recurrent disease distant from the ablation site.

Local control at 1 year was seen in 67%. Kaplan-Meier analysis yielded an actuarial survival of 55% at 2 years postablation and 45% at 3 years postablation.

RADIOFREQUENCY ABLATION

During RFA, a high-frequency electrical current heats and coagulates tissue. This alternating current moves from an active electrode placed within the tumor to dispersive electrodes (Bovie pads) placed on the patient. RFA systems, therefore, have three components: (1) a generator, (2) an active electrode, and (3) a dispersive electrode. As the radiofrequency energy moves from the active electrode to the dispersive electrode and then back to the active electrode, ions within the tissue oscillate to follow the changing direction of the alternating current. This results in frictional heating of the tissue; as the temperature within the tissue rises to greater than 60°C, instantaneous cell death begins because of protein denaturation and coagulation necrosis. Typically, when RFA is performed, the local temperature in the ablated tumor will be 60°C and above.

Like MWA, it is performed under CT guidance using local anesthesia. It leads to necrosis of tumor without significantly affecting the surrounding parenchyma. The so-called "heat-sink" phenomenon is a major limitation. Vessels larger than 3 mm in diameter reduce the amount of energy delivered to the target as a result of the loss of heat through convection within the circulatory system.[40] Other limitations are the size and site of the tumor. Tumors larger than 3 cm usually have a less than 50% necrosis.[41] Also, RFA is prohibitory for central tumors because of the risk of injuries to bronchus, major vessels, and esophagus.

In an earlier report from University of Pittsburgh, Herrera and colleagues[41] reported the results in 18 patients (5 NSCLC and 13 metastasis) treated with RFA. Response, assessed by the modified RECIST criteria, was complete in 6% and partial in 44% of patients. Fernando and colleagues[42] reported the results in 18 patients with NSCLC, of which nine patients were stage I patients. The median follow-up was 14 months and local progression occurred in 38% of nodules. The mean and median progression-free intervals were 16.8 and 17.6 months, respectively. For stage I NSCLC, the mean progression-free interval was 17.6 months and the median progression-free interval was not reached. Subsequently, Pennathur and colleagues[43] reported the results of 19 patients with stage I NSCLC treated with RFA. The mean follow-up was 29 months. Local progression occurred in 42% of patients and the median time to progression was 27 months. The estimated OS at 1 year was 95%.

Gadaleta and colleagues[44] described their preliminary experience in 18 patients (4 NSCLC and 14 metastases). The median follow-up was 8 months and 94% of patients did not have any local progression. Similarly, Yasui and colleagues[45] reported the early results of RFA (median follow-up, 7 months posttreatment) in 99 tumors and saw local progression in only nine tumors. Yan and colleagues[46] reported the results of 55 medically inoperable patients with pulmonary metastases from colorectal neoplasms who were treated with RFA. They reported a median OS of 33 months, and estimated 1-, 2-, and 3-year survivals of 85%, 64%, and 46%, respectively. A local recurrence rate of 38% was reported for these patients.

Ambrogi and colleagues[47] reported the results of RFA in 54 patients with 64 lung lesions (40 NSCLC and 24 metastases). The authors used contrast enhancement on CT scans to assess initial response and used modified RECIST criteria after 6 months to assess the progression of the lesion. They reported a complete response rate of 62%. Mean follow-up was 23.7 months with an OS of 28.9 months. The median progression-free interval was 24.1 months. Another interesting study by Hiraki and colleagues[48] evaluated the risk factors for local progression after RFA in a series of 128 patients with 342 tumors. There were 317 metastatic lesions and 25 primary lung neoplasms; the Boston Scientific (Marlborough, MA) expandable probe was used in 142 lesions and Valley Lab (Medtronic, Dublin, Ireland) cluster probe was used in 200 lesions. The mean follow-up was 12 months and local progression was seen in 94 lesions (27%). Comparing the multitined probe with cooled-tip probe showed that the use of cooled-tip probe was an independent risk factor for local progression.

Lee and colleagues[49] reported their experience in 10 patients with stage I NSCLC. Mean survival was 21 months with 80% of patients being alive at the end of 14.8 months of follow-up. Most recently Lencioni and colleagues[50] reported the results of a prospective, intention-to-treat, single-arm, multicenter clinical trial from seven centers in Europe, the United States, and Australia (RAPTURE TRIAL). RFA was performed in 183 tumors of 106 patients. Malignancy was confirmed by biopsy in all patients. Diagnoses included NSCLC in 33 patients, metastasis from colorectal carcinoma in 53 patients, and metastasis from other primary malignancies in 20 patients. In patients with NSCLC, OS was 70% (95% CI, 51%–83%) at 1 year and 48% (95% CI, 30%–65%) at 2 years. Patients with stage I NSCLC (N = 13) had a 2-year OS of 75% (45%–92%) and a 2-year cancer-specific survival of 92% (66%–99%). In patients with colorectal metastases, OS was 89% (95% CI, 76%–95%) at 1 year and 66% (95% CI, 53%–79%) at 2 years. For patients with other metastases, OS was 92% (95% CI, 65%–99%) at 1 year and 64% (95% CI, 43%–82%) at 2 years.

Results of the ACOSOG Z4033 were recently published.[51] In this randomized multicenter US trial 54 patients with medically inoperable, biopsy proven, stage IA NSCLC were treated with percutaneous CT-guided RFA. The OS rate was 86.3% at 1 year and 69.8% at 2 years. The local tumor recurrence-free rate was 68.9% at 1 year and 59.8% at 2 years and was worse for tumors greater than 2 cm. Nineteen patients had recurrence. There were 21 grade 3 adverse events, two grade 4 adverse events, and one grade 5 adverse event in 12 patients within the first 90 days after RFA. None of the grade 4 or 5 adverse events were attributable to RFA. A tumor size less than 2.0 cm and a performance status of 0 or 1 were associated with statistically significant improved survival of 83% and 78%, respectively, at 2 years.

PATIENT SELECTION

Patients with limited-stage lung cancer and metastatic disease to the lung, who otherwise would have been candidates for surgery but deemed inoperable because of their comorbidities or who choose ablative therapies because of personal preference, are usually candidates for ablative therapies. For NSCLC, ablative therapies can be used for stage I patients who are believed to be at increased risk for any kind of pulmonary resection or who refuse surgery. Occasionally, ablative therapies are a reasonable therapy option for a patient with more advanced cancer. Such patients include those with a second nodule within the same tumor lobe or a satellite nodule within another lobe. This subgroup of advanced-stage tumors may be more appropriately treated with resection, as long as the cancer is localized to the lung. However, in those patients who are believed to be at increased operative risk, ablative therapies are good alternatives. Other patients who may be considered for treatment with these modalities include those with advanced-stage disease who have responded to definitive radiation therapy and chemotherapy but have a persistent, solitary lesion and those who have a recurrent isolated cancer after previous lung resection.

Ablative therapies are also a suitable option for some patients with limited peripheral pulmonary metastases. As with resection, this treatment should be reserved for those patients with a limited number of metastases, disease localized to the chest, and with their primary cancer either controlled or controllable. Situations may also occur where complete resection of all pulmonary metastases is not possible. In these situations, ablation of some nodules may be an alternative intraoperatively or postoperatively.

Combination of Ablative Therapies

A recent study from University of Pittsburgh reported use of SABR for recurrent tumors, including recurrence after MWA and RFA.[52] Similarly, recurrent tumors or local failures after SABR can be treated with either surgery or MWA. Also patients with larger (>4 cm) tumors can be treated with a combination of SABR and MWA for a better complete ablation. This approach can be a basis of a future trial.

SUMMARY

The treatment paradigm for early stage lung cancer and oligometastatic disease to the lung is rapidly changing. Ablative therapies, especially SABR, are challenging the surgical gold standard and have the potential to be the standard for operable patients with early stage lung cancer who are high risk for morbidities. MWA is another promising novel ablative modality that in the near future would also be available for transbronchial ablation of small lung tumors, especially more central tumors. The Z4033 trial shows a 2-year overall survival rate with RFA comparable with SABR. The outcome results of the ablative therapies should be compared with anatomic minimally invasive segmentectomy or lobectomy with lymph node dissection rather than historical surgical data.

REFERENCES

1. Stewart BW, Wild C, editors. World cancer report, 2014. Lyon (France): International Agency for Research on Cancer; World Health Organization; 2014.
2. Bach PB, Cramer LD, Warren JL, et al. Racial differences in the treatment of early stage non-small cell lung cancer. N Engl J Med 1999;341:1198–205.
3. Sibley G, Jamieson T, Marks L, et al. Radiotherapy alone for medically inoperable stage I non-small-cell lung cancer: the Duke experience. Int J Radiat Oncol Biol Phys 1998;40:149–54.
4. Kupelian PA, Komaki R, Allen P. Prognostic factors in the treatment of node-negative non-small cell lung carcinoma with radiation alone. Int J Radiat Oncol Biol Phys 1996;36:607–13.
5. Zierhut D, Bettscheider C, Schubert K, et al. Radiation therapy of stage I and II non-small cell lung cancer. Lung Cancer 2001;34:S39–43.
6. Abratt RP, Morgan GW. Lung toxicity following chest irradiation in patients with lung cancer. Lung Cancer 2002;35:103–9.
7. Byhardt RW, Martin L, Pajak TF, et al. The influence of field size and other treatment factors on pulmonary toxicity following hyperfractionated irradiation for inoperable non-small cell lung cancer (NSCLC): analysis of a Radiation Therapy Oncology Group (RTOG) protocol. Int J Radiat Oncol Biol Phys 1993;27:537–44.
8. Bradley J, Graham MV, Winter K, et al. Toxicity and outcome results of RTOG 9311: a phase I-II dose-escalation study using three-dimensional conformal radiotherapy in patients with inoperable non-small-cell lung carcinoma. Int J Radiat Oncol Biol Phys 2005;61:318–28.

9. Kong FM, Hayman JA, Griffith KA, et al. Final toxicity results of a radiation-dose escalation study in patients with non-small-cell lung cancer (NSCLC): predictors for radiation pneumonitis and fibrosis. Int J Radiat Oncol Biol Phys 2006;65(4): 1075–86.

10. Fernando HC, Abbas G. Alternatives to surgical resection for non-small cell lung cancer. In: Pearson FG, Patterson GA, editors. Pearson's thoracic & esophageal surgery. Philadelphia: Churchill Livingstone/Elsevier; 2008. p. 796–803.

11. Douglas BG, Fowler JF. The effect of multiple small doses of x rays on skin reactions in the mouse and a basic interpretation. Radiat Res 1976;66:401–26.

12. Fowler JF, Tome WA, Fenwick JD, et al. A challenge to traditional radiation oncology. Int J Radiat Oncol Biol Phys 2004;60:1241–56.

13. McGarry RC, Papiez L, Williams M, et al. Stereotactic body radiation therapy of early-stage non small-cell lung carcinoma: phase I study. Int J Radiat Oncol Biol Phys 2005;63:1010–5.

14. Timmerman R, McGarry R, Yiannoutsos C, et al. Excessive toxicity when treating central tumors in a phase II study of stereotactic body radiation therapy for medically inoperable early-stage lung cancer. J Clin Oncol 2006;24:4833–9.

15. Timmerman R, Paulus R, Galvin J, et al. Stereotactic body radiation therapy for inoperable early stage lung cancer. JAMA 2010;303:1070–6.

16. Timmerman RD, Hu C, Michalski J, et al. Long-term results of RTOG 0236: a phase II trial of stereotactic body radiation therapy (SBRT) in the treatment of patients with medically inoperable stage I non small cell lung cancer. Int J Radiat Oncol Biol Phys 2014;90(Suppl):S30.

17. Pennathur A, Luketich JD, Heron DE, et al. Stereotactic radiosurgery for the treatment of lung neoplasm: experience in 100 consecutive patients. Ann Thorac Surg 2009;88(5):1594–600.

18. Pennathur A, Luketich JD, Heron DE, et al. Stereotactic radiosurgery for the treatment of stage I non small cell lung cancer in high risk patients. J Thorac Cardiovasc Surg 2009;137(3):597–604.

19. Pennathur A, Luketich JD, Heron DE, et al. Stereotactic radiotherapy/stereotactic body radiotherapy for recurrent lung neoplasm: an analysis of outcome in 100 patients. Ann Thorac Surg 2015;100(6):2019–24.

20. Onishi H, Shirato H, Nagata Y, et al. Hypofractionated stereotactic radiotherapy (HypoFXSRT) for stage I non small cell lung cancer: updated results of 257 patients in a Japanese multi-institutional study. J Thorac Oncol 2007;2(7 Suppl 3): S94–100.

21. Nagata Y, Takayama K, Matsuo Y, et al. Clinical outcomes of a phase I/II study of 48 Gy of stereotactic body radiotherapy in 4 fractions for primary lung cancer using a stereotactic body frame. Int J Radiat Oncol Biol Phys 2005;63:1427–31.

22. Nagata Y, Hiraoka M, Shibata T, et al. A phase II trial of stereotactic body radiation therapy for operable T1N0M0 non–small cell lung cancer: Japan Clinical Oncology Group (JCOG0403). Int J Radiat Oncol Biol Phys 2010;78(Suppl): S27–8.

23. Nagata Y, Hiraoka M, Shibata T, et al. Prospective trial of stereotactic body radiation therapy for both operable and in-operable T1N0M0 non small cell lung cancer. Int J Radiat Oncol Biol Phys 2015;93(5):989–96.

24. Timmerman RD, Paulus R, Pass HI, et al. RTOG 0618: Stereotactic body radiation therapy (SBRT) to treat operable early-stage lung cancer patients. J Clin Oncol 2013;31:abstr 7523.

25. Videtic GM, Hu C, Singh AK, et al. A randomized phase 2 study comparing 2 stereotactic body radiation therapy schedules for medically inoperable patients with

stage I peripheral non small cell lung cancer: NRG Oncology RTOG 0915. Int J Radiat Oncol Biol Phys 2015;93(4):757–64.

26. Crabtree TD, Denlinger CE, Meyers BF, et al. Stereotactic body radiation therapy versus surgical resection for stage I non-small cell lung cancer. J Thorac Cardiovasc Surg 2010;140:377–86.

27. Verstegen NE, Oosterhuis JW, Palma DA, et al. Stage I-II non-small-cell lung cancer treated using either stereotactic ablative radiotherapy (SABR) or lobectomy by video-assisted thoracoscopic surgery (VATS): outcomes of a propensity score-matched analysis. Ann Oncol 2013;24:1543–8.

28. Mokhles S, Verstegen N, Maat AP, et al. Comparison of clinical outcome of stage I non-small cell lung cancer treated surgically or with stereotactic radiotherapy: results from propensity score analysis. Lung Cancer 2015;87:283–9.

29. Van den Berg LL, Klinkenberg TJ, Groen HJ, et al. Patterns of recurrence and survival after surgery or stereotactic radiotherapy for early stage NSCLC. J Thorac Oncol 2015;10:826–31.

30. Shirvani SM, Jiang J, Chang JY, et al. Comparative effectiveness of 5 treatment strategies for early-stage non-small cell lung cancer in the elderly. Int J Radiat Oncol Biol Phys 2012;84:1060–70.

31. Shirvani SM, Jiang J, Chang JY, et al. Lobectomy, sublobar resection, and stereotactic ablative radiotherapy for early-stage non-small cell lung cancers in the elderly. JAMA Surg 2014;149:1244–53.

32. Chang JY, Senan S, Paul MA, et al. Stereotactic ablative radiotherapy versus lobectomy for operable stage I non-small-cell lung cancer: a pooled analysis of two randomised trials. Lancet Oncol 2015;16:630–7.

33. Okada M, Yoshikawa K, Hatta T, et al. Is segmentectomy with lymph node assessment an alternative to lobectomy for non small cell lung cancer of 2 cm or smaller? Ann Thorac Surg 2001;71:956–60.

34. Schuchert MJ, Abbas G, Awais O, et al. Anatomic segmentectomy for the solitary pulmonary nodule and early-stage lung cancer. Ann Thorac Surg 2012;93(6): 1780–5 [discussion: 1786–7].

35. Landreneau RJ, Normolle DP, Christie NA, et al. Recurrence and survival outcomes after anatomic segmentectomy versus lobectomy for clinical stage I non-small-cell lung cancer: a propensity-matched analysis. J Clin Oncol 2014; 32(23):2449–55.

36. Crabtree T, Puri V, Timmerman R, et al. Treatment of stage I lung cancer in high-risk and inoperable patients: comparison of prospective clinical trials using stereotactic body radiotherapy (RTOG 0236), sublobar resection (ACOSOG Z4032), and radiofrequency ablation (ACOSOG Z4033). J Thorac Cardiovasc Surg 2013;145(3):692–9.

37. Feng W, Liu W, Liu C, et al. Percutaneous microwave coagulation therapy for lung cancer. Zhonghua Zhong Liu Za Zhi 2002;24:388–90.

38. Simon CS, Dupuy DE, Mayo-Smith WW. Microwave ablation: principles and applications. Radiographics 2005;25:S69–83.

39. Wolf FJ, Grand DJ, Machan JT, et al. Microwave ablation of lung malignancies: effectiveness, CT findings, and safety in 50 patients. Radiology 2008;247(3): 871–9.

40. Lencioni R, Crocetti L, Cioni R, et al. Radiofrequency ablation of lung malignancies: where do we stand? Cardiovasc Intervent Radiol 2004;27:581–90.

41. Herrera LJ, Fernando HC, Perry Y, et al. Radiofrequency ablation of pulmonary malignant tumors in nonsurgical candidates. J Thorac Cardiovasc Surg 2003; 125(4):929–37.

42. Fernando HC, De Hoyos A, Landreneau RJ, et al. Radiofrequency ablation for the treatment of non-small cell lung cancer in marginal surgical candidates. J Thorac Cardiovasc Surg 2005;129:261–7.

43. Pennathur A, Luketich JD, Abbas G, et al. Radiofrequency ablation of stage I non-small cell lung neoplasm. J Thorac Cardiovasc Surg 2007;134:857–64.

44. Gadaleta C, Mattioli V, Colucci G, et al. Radiofrequency ablation of 40 lung neoplasms preliminary results. Am J Roentgenol 2004;183:361–9.

45. Yasui K, Kanazawa S, Sano Y, et al. Thoracic tumors treated with CT-guided radiofrequency ablation: initial experience. Radiology 2004;231(3):850–7.

46. Yan TD, King J, Sjarif A, et al. Percutaneous radiofrequency ablation of pulmonary metastases from colorectal carcinoma: prognostic determinants for survival. Ann Surg Oncol 2006;13(11):1529–37.

47. Ambrogi MC, Lucchi M, Dini P, et al. Percutaneous radiofrequency ablation of lung tumors: results in mid term. Eur J Cardiothorac Surg 2006;30(1):177–83.

48. Hiraki T, Sakuraj J, Tsuda T, et al. Risk factors for local progression after percutaneous radiofrequency ablation of lung tumors: evaluation based on a preliminary review of 342 patients. Cancer 2006;107(12):2873–80.

49. Lee JM, Jin GY, Goldber SN, et al. Percutaneous radiofrequency ablation of lung neoplasms: initial therapeutic response. Radiology 2004;230:125–34.

50. Lencioni R, Crocetti L, Cioni R, et al. Response to radiofrequency ablation of pulmonary tumors: a prospective, intention-to-treat, multicentre clinical trial (the RAPTURE study). Lancet Oncol 2008;9(7):621–8.

51. Dupuy DE, Fernando HC, Hillman S, et al. Radiofrequency ablation of stage IA non-small cell lung cancer in medically inoperable patients: results from the American College of Surgeons Oncology Group Z4033 (Alliance) trial. Cancer 2015;121(19):3491–8.

52. Pennathur A, Luketich JD, Heron DE, et al. Stereotactic radiosurgery/stereotactic body radiotherapy for recurrent lung neoplasm: an analysis of outcomes in 100 patients. Ann Thorac Surg 2015;100(6):2019–24.

Neoadjuvant Therapy in Non–Small Cell Lung Cancer

Yifan Zheng, MD, Michael T. Jaklitsch, MD, Raphael Bueno, MD*

KEYWORDS

- Stage IIIA non–small cell lung cancer (NSCLC) • N2 nodal disease • Stage IIIA(N2)
- Neoadjuvant concurrent therapy • Preoperative therapy • Chemotherapy
- Radiation therapy • Lung cancer

KEY POINTS

- A complete evaluation of patients diagnosed with lung cancer should include a comprehensive medical history, physical examination, analysis of functional capacity, relevant imaging studies, pathological studies, and a discussion about the patients' goals.
- A review of the tumor subtype and pathologic assessment of the lymph nodes enables the assignment of the most accurate clinical stage.
- Neoadjuvant chemoradiation is used to treat patients with resectable, locally advanced NSCLC with the following goals:
  - Eliminate micrometastatic systemic disease
  - Prevent tumor growth, achieve downstaging, and sterilize affected lymph nodes
  - Provide time for an oncologic stress test, ensuring that during treatment, metastatic disease does not appear.
- The current recommended preoperative regimen is a concurrent platinum-based chemotherapy course with 54 Gy of thoracic radiation.
- After surgery, the pathologic stage can be informative as to prognosis and any need for additional therapy; after trimodality therapy, patients should have a regular follow-up with tobacco abstinence support and recurrence/metastasis screening.

INTRODUCTION

Lung cancer remains the leading cause of cancer death worldwide.[1] It is quite heterogeneous and is subdivided into small cell lung cancer (20%) and non–small cell lung cancer (NSCLC), with the latter affecting 80% of patients. NSCLC itself is composed

The authors have nothing to disclose.
Division of Thoracic Surgery, Brigham and Women's Hospital, Harvard Medical School, 75 Francis Street, Boston, MA 02115, USA
* Corresponding author.
E-mail address: rbueno@partners.org

Surg Oncol Clin N Am 25 (2016) 567–584
http://dx.doi.org/10.1016/j.soc.2016.02.010
1055-3207/16/$ – see front matter © 2016 Elsevier Inc. All rights reserved.

of several types, including adenocarcinoma, squamous cell carcinoma, large cell carcinoma, and neuroendocrine tumors. In each of these histologic subtypes, cancer stage has a significant impact on the prognosis.

According to the International Association for the Study of Lung Cancer Staging Project, the overall 5-year survival for stage IA NSCLC is 66%, stage IB is 56%, stage IIA is 43%, stage IIB is 35%, and stage IIIA is 23%.[2] Five-year survivals for stages IIIB and IV disease are lower than 10%.[3] Treatment of NSCLC includes chemotherapy, radiation, and/or surgery, with different combinations and order of therapies depending on the stage of the disease. The steps of evaluating patients with suspected lung cancer, the current neoadjuvant therapies, and the evaluation of the therapeutic effect are reviewed herein.

DEFINITION OF NEOADJUVANT THERAPY

Neoadjuvant therapy is defined as either chemotherapy or radiotherapy given before the surgical excision of a malignant tumor. It often involves a combination of both treatment modalities, and it is used to treat some patients with locally advanced stages of NSCLC who have good performance status. Neoadjuvant therapy is given with the intent of

1. Eradicating N2 nodal disease.
2. Eliminating micrometastatic systemic disease.
3. Controlling the tumor in intermediate stage lung cancer to provide a time period to ascertain that patients are not harboring metastatic disease that will appear after surgery.
4. Sufficiently reducing the extent of tumor to enable a lesser resection (eg, converting a pneumonectomy to a lobectomy).

There may be better drug delivery of chemotherapy before alteration of vascular supply to the primary tumor during surgery. Another consideration is that a substantial number of patients are not able to complete adjuvant therapy after undergoing extensive surgery; giving chemotherapy upfront is more likely to provide access for both therapies to a larger number of patients.[4] Finally, giving chemoradiotherapy preoperatively allows for the assessment of the effect at surgery. This judgment of efficacy is not possible if chemoradiotherapy is given postoperatively, after the tumor has been completely removed.

Like all other therapies, neoadjuvant therapy is not without its risks. Disease can progress during neoadjuvant treatment, and some patients may never undergo surgery. Functional status can decline as a result of adverse reactions to therapy, delaying surgery. Neoadjuvant radiation therapy is also associated with scarring and can increase the risk of needing larger pulmonary resections (pneumonectomy).

EARLY STUDIES ON NEOADJUVANT THERAPY

The results of several prospective phase II clinical trials have demonstrated that neoadjuvant therapy is effective in downstaging NSCLC, with some studies reporting an increase in the length of survival.[4–7] In 1992, Strauss and colleagues[5] completed a phase II study evaluating the response of patients with stage IIIA NSCLC to concurrent neoadjuvant cisplatin/vinblastine/fluorouracil and radiation therapy followed by surgery and adjuvant radiation therapy. As one of the first trials with trimodality therapy, this study showed that 66% of the patients had a complete clinical response to neoadjuvant chemoradiation and 17% had a partial response. Thirty-one of 41 patients in the study underwent surgery, and 25 patients had surgical resection. Trimodality therapy was demonstrated to be effective, but there was substantial treatment toxicity in this study with a 15% (6 deaths) treatment-related mortality rate and only modest improvement in median length of survival to 15.5 months.

The Southwest Oncology Group (SWOG) 8805 study by Albain and colleagues[7] also evaluated trimodality therapy with cisplatin and etoposide, radiotherapy, and surgery (or additional chemotherapy and radiation instead of surgery for unresectable disease) in patients with stage IIIA(N2) and IIIB(N2/N3) disease. This study reported encouraging survival rates, particularly for patients with no residual N2 disease at surgery. The median survival was 30 months for patients with no residual N2 disease versus 9 months for patients with residual N2 disease ($P = .002$). A multicenter phase II study by Sugarbaker and colleagues[4] in 1995 (Cancer and Leukemia Group B [CALGB] 8935) assessed the effectiveness of neoadjuvant cisplatin and vinblastine followed by surgery and adjuvant chemotherapy and radiation (54 Gy) for complete resection or followed by 59.4 Gy of radiation after incomplete/no resection in patients with stage IIIA(N2) NSCLC. This study reported longer lengths of median survival for patients able to undergo complete resection as compared with those with incomplete resection or no resection (20.9 months vs 17.8 months vs 8.5 months, respectively).

In addition to demonstrating a therapeutic effect, both the SWOG 8805 and CALGB 8935 studies reported lower mortality rates than previous studies: 13 (10.0%) and 4 (5.4%) treatment-related deaths, respectively. Of the 13 patients in the SWOG 8805 study, 5 died preoperatively and 8 died postoperatively (5 had intrapericardial pneumonectomy, 1 had a standard pneumonectomy, and 2 had lobectomies). In the CALGB 8935 study, 1 patient died preoperatively, 2 died postoperatively, and 1 died during treatment with adjuvant chemotherapy. Along with lower mortality rates, these studies also reported acceptable morbidity rates, demonstrating better treatment tolerance.

In 1994, single-center phase III studies compared neoadjuvant chemotherapy followed by surgery with surgery alone. The study by Rosell and colleagues[8] compared patients with stage IIIA(N0-2) NSCLC treated with neoadjuvant mitomycin/ifosfamide/cisplatin, surgery, and adjuvant radiation with those treated with surgery and adjuvant radiation. This study found an improved median survival of 26 months versus 8 months, in favor of treatment with neoadjuvant chemotherapy ($P<.001$). Roth and colleagues[9] conducted a similar study comparing treatment with neoadjuvant cyclophosphamide/etoposide/cisplatin followed by surgery and adjuvant chemotherapy with surgery alone in patients with stage IIIA(N0-2) NSCLC. This study also reported an improved median survival of 64 months versus 8 months, in favor of neoadjuvant chemotherapy treatment ($P<.008$).

The benefit seen in prognostic improvement is likely due to downstaged disease, specifically, eradication of nodal disease. A retrospective review in 2000 evaluating the outcomes of 103 patients who underwent surgery after neoadjuvant therapy for stage IIIA(N2) NSCLC found that patients whose nodal disease was eradicated had significantly improved 35.8% 5-year survival compared with patients with persistent N1 and N2 nodal disease who had a 9% 5-year survival.[10] Four patients died within 30 days of surgery, 2 of whom underwent pneumonectomies and 2 of whom underwent lobectomies. Analysis of nodal status after neoadjuvant therapy followed by surgery in the CALGB 8935 study also found that those patients with persistent N2 cancer had significantly decreased failure-free survival (median failure-free survival 8.2 months vs 47.8 months in patients with no residual N2 disease, $P = .01$).[6] Therefore, the major goal for treating patients with neoadjuvant therapy for stage IIIA(N2) NSCLC became focused on eliminating nodal disease.

NEOADJUVANT THERAPY VERSUS ADJUVANT THERAPY

The SWOG S9900 phase III study evaluated neoadjuvant carboplatin and paclitaxel with surgery versus surgery alone in treating patients with stage IB, II, or select IIIA NSCLC (no superior sulcus tumors or tumors with N2 disease).[11] The overall survival and progression-free survival was improved with neoadjuvant chemotherapy as compared with surgery alone (overall survival: median 62 months vs 41 months, respectively; progression-free survival: 33 months vs 20 months, respectively), but these results did not reach statistical significance. Furthermore, this study closed early after results were published demonstrating the nonsignificant but intriguing survival benefit from adjuvant therapy in patients with early stage NSCLC.

In 2003, a Japanese phase III study compared patients with completely resected stage I and II NSCLC who were treated with adjuvant uracil and tegafur versus those treated with surgery alone.[12] No survival benefits were observed with the addition of the adjuvant regimen becauase the overall 5-year survival rate was found to be 79% for the adjuvant group and 75% for the control group (not statistically significant) and the disease-free survival rate was 78% and 71%, respectively (also not statistically significant). These survivals are higher than other reports and may represent a study of homogeneous early stage NSCLC tumors.

Alternatively, the International Adjuvant Lung Cancer Trial was a phase III trial that compared treating early stage NSCLC with postoperative cisplatin therapy versus observation and found that patients treated with adjuvant chemotherapy had significantly higher 5-year overall survival (44.5% vs 40.4%, hazard ratio [HR] 0.86, 95% confidence interval [CI] 0.76–0.98, $P<.03$) and disease-free survival (39.4% vs 34.3%, HR 0.83, 95% CI 0.74–0.94, $P<.003$).[13] These lower survival rates may reflect a larger population of participants with occult, higher-stage disease. The National Cancer Institute of Canada Clinical Trials Group JBR.10 trial was a phase III study that also reported significantly improved overall survival (94 vs 73 months, HR 0.69, $P = .04$) and disease-free survival (not reached vs 46.7 months, HR 0.60, $P<.001$) in patients with completely resected stage IB and II NSCLC who were treated with adjuvant vinorelbine and cisplatin versus observation.[14] However, when the survival data on the subgroup with stage IB disease were analyzed, no significant benefit was associated with adjuvant chemotherapy. The Cancer and Leukemia Group B 9633 phase III trial specifically studied patients with stage I NSCLC and found that the only statistically significant survival advantage to adjuvant paclitaxel and carboplatin as compared with observation was seen in patients with tumors 4 cm or greater in diameter (HR 0.69, 95% CI 0.48–0.99, $P = .043$).[15]

A prospective randomized trial by the Spanish Lung Cancer Group compared 3 treatment arms in 624 patients with early stage NSCLC: 201 patients underwent treatment with preoperative chemotherapy plus surgery (preoperative); 211 patients underwent treatment with surgery plus adjuvant chemotherapy (adjuvant); and 212 patients had surgery alone (control).[16] Chemotherapies given either preoperatively or in the adjuvant setting were 3 cycles of paclitaxel (200 mg/m^2 intravenously [IV] over 3 hours) and carboplatin (area under the curve dose of 6 mg/mL/min IV over 30–60 minutes). The results of this trial found that there was no statistically significant difference in the 5-year disease-free survival between the preoperative and control arms (38.3% vs 34.1%, HR 0.92, $P = .176$) or between the adjuvant and control arms (36.6% vs 34.1%, HR 0.96, $P = .74$). The overall survival at 5-year was 46.6%, 45.5%, and 44.0% for the preoperative, adjuvant, and control arms, respectively, with no significant difference across the treatment arms.

The Spanish Lung Cancer Group study did not demonstrate that the addition of chemotherapy to surgery, either preoperatively or postoperatively, would improve disease-free survival; but the study was likely limited by the inclusion of a large number of patients with stage I NSCLC (74.3%, 77.6%, and 73.3% of the preoperative, adjuvant, and control cohorts, respectively). However, the investigators did note an advantage of giving chemotherapy preoperatively as opposed to postoperatively. They concluded that because the treatment decision was made before surgery by the randomization, more patients were able to receive chemotherapy preoperatively. Given that the percentage of patients who started chemotherapy preoperatively (97.0%) versus the percentage that began therapy in the adjuvant arm (66.2%) was higher, this study seems to indicate that chemotherapy may be better tolerated in a neoadjuvant setting.

A meta-analysis of the results of 15 randomized controlled trials showed that neoadjuvant chemotherapy provided a 13% reduction in the relative risk of death (HR 0.87, 95% CI 0.78–0.96, $P = .007$), which represents an absolute survival improvement of 5% at 5 years (40% to 45%) for patients with resectable stage IB to IIIA NSCLC, regardless of the chemotherapy regimen (most were platinum based).[17] The same study also found that recurrence-free survival (HR 0.85, 95% CI 0.76–0.94, $P = .002$) and time to distant recurrence (HR 0.69, 95% CI 0.58–0.82, $P<.0001$) was improved by preoperative chemotherapy. These findings show that neoadjuvant chemotherapy followed by surgery is an effective treatment approach, particularly for locally advanced disease.

Studies have also addressed the sequence in which to give radiation therapy in the multimodality treatment of NSCLC. A phase III study by the German Lung Cancer Cooperative Group (GLCCG) compared treatment with cisplatin and etoposide, then concurrent radiation and carboplatin and vindesine, followed by surgery (intervention group) to treatment with cisplatin and etoposide followed by surgery and adjuvant radiation (control group) in patients with stage IIIA and IIIB NSCLC.[18] A similar number of patients in the intervention (142 patients of 264 eligible) and control (154 patients of 260 eligible) groups were able to undergo surgery and a similar number in either group had complete resection (98 and 84, respectively). Of the patients who had a complete resection, the ones receiving neoadjuvant chemoradiation were more likely to have a pathologic response (60% vs 20%, $P<.0001$) and mediastinal downstaging (46% vs 29%, $P = .02$). Although the overall survival and progression-free survival were not significantly different between both groups, neoadjuvant radiation was proven effective for decreasing disease burden to allow for a lesser resection.

PATIENT EVALUATION OVERVIEW

Early stage NSCLC includes stage I and II cancer and is treated with surgical resection. Current practice standards are to evaluate patients with resected stage IB tumors 4 cm or greater or stage II disease for postoperative chemotherapy and potential clinical trials. Patients with a higher risk of recurrence based on features, such as lymphovascular invasion, poor tumor differentiation, and potentially unfavorable molecular prognostic tests, may also be considered for adjuvant chemotherapy.[19] Neoadjuvant and adjuvant radiation are currently not recommended for stage I and II NSCLC unless the goals are to downstage the tumor to allow for a lesser resection or to sterilize positive margins. A study by Wang and colleagues[20] found that postoperative radiotherapy is associated with improved overall survival in patients with incomplete resection of their stage II or III(N0-2) tumor.

Table 1
Current standards of treatment of non–small cell lung cancer by clinical stage (American Joint Committee on Cancer Staging Manual, 7th Edition)

	Description[22]	Treatment[23]
Stage I	T1a-2aN0M0	Surgical resection (lobectomy vs sublobar resection based on size/location)
		Consider SBRT for medically inoperable patients or patients who decline surgery
		Consider adjuvant therapy for tumors >4 cm in diameter[15]
Stage II	T1a-3N0-1M0	Surgical resection
		Consider concurrent chemoradiation for medically inoperable patients
		Consider adjuvant therapy
Stage IIIA	T1a-4N0-2M0	*Neoadjuvant therapy*
		Restaging (lack of downstaging may warrant definitive chemoradiotherapy rather than proceeding to surgery)
		Surgical resection
		Consider adjuvant therapy
Stage IIIB	T1a-4N2-3M0	Neoadjuvant therapy in select cases, chemotherapy, radiation therapy, palliative surgery in special circumstances
Stage IV	T1a-4N0-3M1a-b	Chemotherapy, radiation therapy, palliative surgery (no neoadjuvant therapy)

Abbreviation: SBRT, stereotactic body radiation therapy.

Neoadjuvant concurrent chemoradiation is a part of the standard treatment of resectable stage IIIA NSCLC (and select cases of localized IIIB disease).[7,11,21] Adjuvant therapy is also considered in the postoperative management of these patients. Advanced disease, which includes stages IIIB and IV NSCLC, is usually treated with definitive or palliative chemotherapy with or without radiation therapy. There are special cases of advanced disease, such as local invasion of the trachea, esophagus, blood vessels, heart or spine, or oligometastatic disease affecting the brain or adrenal gland, that can be technically resected. Adjuvant therapy should also be considered after surgical resection in these cases (**Table 1**).

Specific Indications for Neoadjuvant Therapy

The current clinical standard for the treatment of resectable stage IIIA NSCLC is neoadjuvant chemotherapy with/without concurrent radiation therapy, followed by surgical resection, and with/without adjuvant therapy. Stage IIIA disease is a heterogeneous category. It consists of tumors with metastasis to the ipsilateral mediastinal or subcarinal lymph nodes. The primary tumor may have invaded the parietal pleura, the chest wall, the diaphragm, or the main bronchus. A stage IIIA NSCLC tumor can also have no mediastinal lymph node metastasis but have invasion into other mediastinal structures, the great vessels, the carina/trachea, or a vertebral body; alternatively, it may consist of 2 or more tumor nodules in separate ipsilateral lobes. Mediastinal nodal involvement in NSCLC (stage IIIA[N2]) is associated with a worse outcome.[10] Patients with stage IIIA disease are at higher risk than patients with early stage NSCLC for both local tumor progression and occult metastases. Thus, the disease management must be designed to treat both local and metastatic disease. No studies to date definitively prove the superiority of using neoadjuvant chemotherapy versus neoadjuvant chemoradiation. The National Comprehensive Cancer Network's

(NCCN) recommendation is for neoadjuvant chemotherapy to treat metastatic disease and concurrent neoadjuvant radiation to treat local disease.[23]

Nonbulky stage IIIA disease is defined as involving only one lymph node station and a small lymph node size, such as less than 3 cm, or the likely presence of microscopic disease (not detected preoperatively). Bulky disease refers to metastatic disease in multiple mediastinal lymph node stations and large lymph nodes. In 2007, the American College of Chest Physicians (ACCP) conducted a literature search focusing on randomized trials treating stage IIIA NSCLC and concluded that neoadjuvant therapy followed by surgery for known stage IIIA disease is not recommended.[24] They instead recommended combination chemoradiotherapy for all stage IIIA NSCLC with all extents of mediastinal lymph node involvement at preoperative evaluation. However, the trial results available at the time were limited by significant study population heterogeneity, a lack of randomization, or a lack of reliable pretreatment staging. The 3-stage American Joint Committee on Cancer staging system that existed before 1990 was less prognostically accurate,[25] often limited by the prior inclusion of T3N0 with T1-2N2 cancers in the stage IIIA category. Additionally, less emphasis was placed on obtaining a pathologic confirmation of suspected mediastinal nodal disease, and the radiographic imaging used was not sensitive or specific enough for accurate staging of the disease.

In contrast, the guidelines recommended by the NCCN since 2010 support the use of chemoradiation for bulky mediastinal disease but recommend surgery for those patients with single-station N2 disease involvement who respond to neoadjuvant chemotherapy.[26] This NCCN guideline is supported by studies that reported different survival outcomes for patients with bulky nodal disease versus nonbulky nodal disease. In 2000, a retrospective review was conducted by Andre and colleagues[27] of 702 patients with stage IIIA(N2) NSCLC who underwent surgical resection. This study reported that there are subgroups, including clinically detected N2 disease (bulky) and minimal N2 disease (nonbulky, not detected preoperatively), which have different prognoses. Patients who had clinically detectable N2 disease had 5-year survival rates of 18% when treated with preoperative chemotherapy compared with 5% without preoperative chemotherapy ($P<.0001$). The 5-year overall survival rates for patients with clinically detectable N2 disease versus those with minimal N2 disease was 7% and 29%, respectively, when both groups of patients were treated with surgery alone ($P<.0001$, in multivariate analysis). This finding indicated that the extent of mediastinal lymph node involvement should be considered in the treatment of stage IIIA(N2) NSCLC and that different multimodality therapy regimens may be used depending on the stage IIIA disease subgroup.

Bulky disease can also refer to a large primary tumor burden (T3/T4). The phase II SWOG 9416 trial found that the combined modalities of induction chemoradiation (cisplatin and etoposide) and surgical resection led to high rates of complete resection and pathologic complete response in a particular subset of patients with stage IIIA(T3-4N0-1) NSCLC: those with superior sulcus tumors.[28] High rates of complete response or minimal microscopic disease were observed (56% of resection specimens), with better survival in patients with pathologic complete response as compared with survival in patients with residual disease ($P = .02$). These tumors are difficult to resect because they involve the brachial plexus, vertebral bodies, or subclavian vasculature. Neoadjuvant therapy can improve the prognosis of patients with superior sulcus tumors by improving the likelihood of complete surgical resection (**Box 1**).

In select patients with limited IIIA disease and completely resectable metastatic subaortic or para-aortic lymph nodes (station 5 or 6 lymph nodes), surgical resection without induction therapy may be followed by adjuvant therapy; but these instances

---

Box 1
Indications for neoadjuvant therapy followed by surgery

- Stage IIIA NSCLC
  - Nonbulky N2: single-station lymph node disease, small lymph node size
  - Bulky N2: multi-station lymph node disease, large lymph nodes that demonstrate downstaged response to induction chemotherapy and radiation
- Select superior sulcus tumors that involve the brachial plexus/vertebral bodies/subclavian vasculature

---

are rare.[29] There are also recent data to support improved 5-year disease-free survival rates using neoadjuvant therapy to treat patients with stage IIIA(N1) disease (36.6% with preoperative chemotherapy, 31.0% with adjuvant chemotherapy, and 25.0% with surgery alone).[16] In select patients with large IIIB (T4) tumors or minimally involved N3 metastasis, neoadjuvant therapy may downstage the disease to permit surgical resection; but this is not a treatment standard and is still being evaluated in clinical trials.[11,21] These exceptions are beyond the scope of this review.

Staging and Evaluation

Patients presenting with a suspicious lung nodule should undergo a medical interview, a physical examination, and a radiographic and pathologic staging evaluation to determine the optimal treatment regimen. Often the nodule was discovered incidentally on chest radiograph, and patients should undergo a chest computed tomography (CT) evaluation to determine if the nodule has malignant features, such as spiculations. If the clinical and radiologic evaluations are suspicious for cancer, a biopsy of the nodule should be taken, either via CT image-guided fine-needle aspiration or via transbronchial biopsy with guidance by endobronchial ultrasonography (EBUS). Alternatively, a biopsy may be obtained via minimally invasive or open surgery if less invasive biopsies cannot be performed or if the suspicion for cancer is very high.

Staging begins with the chest CT scan, which is used to determine the tumor size and the extent of tumor invasion into nearby structures. Patients also undergo a PET/CT scan to evaluate for metastatic disease in mediastinal lymph nodes and other extrapulmonary sites. If there is suspicion for mediastinal involvement or if the primary tumor is large or centrally located, cervical mediastinoscopy or an EBUS transbronchial biopsy is performed for tissue diagnosis of the metastasis. Organ-specific symptoms or high-stage disease may prompt studies, such as brain MRI, to evaluate for distant metastases. Patients are then given a clinical stage based on the tumor (T), the lymph node (N), and the distant metastatic (M) evaluations and stratified to the most appropriate treatment course.

An important factor to consider in deciding disease management is patients' performance status. Good scores on the Karnofsky Performance Status Scale or the Eastern Cooperative Oncology Group Performance Scale are associated with better tolerance of treatment and less postoperative morbidity. Some studies have also determined that these performance scales have prognostic predictability.[30–32] Before the administration of any neoadjuvant therapy, an assessment of the patients' functional status is performed with one of these scales; the score is considered when choosing the treatment regimen.

CHEMOTHERAPY

The aim of neoadjuvant chemotherapy is to treat micrometastatic disease with a systemic treatment before surgery in order to improve prognosis. Platinum-based chemotherapies are the most commonly used drugs, with studies demonstrating favorable survival results.[33] Platinum drugs are often paired with topoisomerase inhibitors or taxanes for broader antitumor effect.

Preferred neoadjuvant chemotherapy regimens are cisplatin and etoposide or carboplatin and paclitaxel, administered with a concurrent course of radiotherapy. If patients are unable to tolerate cisplatin because of renal insufficiency or hearing loss (adverse effects of cisplatin), carboplatin and paclitaxel may be substituted. A platinum drug and pemetrexed may also be effective, but this regimen is reserved for nonsquamous histologies. Pemetrexed is less effective in squamous cell carcinoma because of a higher expression of thymidylate synthase[34,35] **(Table 2)**.

These full-dose chemotherapy regimens are as recommended by the NCCN. The area under the plasma concentration time curve (AUC) quantifies a given chemotherapy's concentration in the body at a given time after a dose administration. The dose of carboplatin is expressed as an AUC value because the desired serum concentration needs to be adequately controlled for patients with impaired renal function. The target AUC is achieved by accounting for the glomerular filtration rate.

RADIOTHERAPY

The aim of neoadjuvant radiotherapy is to provide local disease control by decreasing the size of the primary tumor. A prospective randomized study by the Radiation Therapy Oncology Group (RTOG) in 1980 compared split and continuous radiation therapy courses as well as treatment with total radiation dosages of 40, 50, or 60 Gy in patients diagnosed with inoperable NSCLC.[40] This study found that the radiation dosages were safe and that patients had a higher survival rate with continuous radiation therapy. Those treated with radiation doses at 50 or 60 Gy had better tumor control than those treated with 40 Gy.

In 2005, a retrospective cohort study compared patients with stage IIIA(N2) NSCLC undergoing surgery after being treated with low-dose (median 45 Gy) radiation with those treated with high-dose (median 60 Gy) radiation.[41] Complete pathologic response was 10% in the low-dose group compared with 28% in the high-dose group ($P = .04$); both groups of therapy were found to be safe with similar morbidity and mortality rates. More recently, a retrospective review of 1041 patients with stage IIIA

Table 2		
Common neoadjuvant chemotherapy regimens and their schedules of administration		
Chemotherapies	**Dose of Administration**	**Frequency of Administration**
Cisplatin and etoposide[7]	Cisplatin 50 mg/m² IV Etoposide 50 mg/m² IV	Day 1, 8, 29, 36 Day 1–5, 29–33
Carboplatin and paclitaxel[36]	Carboplatin AUC 6 mg/mL/min IV over 30 min Paclitaxel 200 mg/m² IV over 3 h	Every 3 wk × 2 cycles
Cisplatin and vinblastine[37]	Cisplatin 100 mg/m² IV Vinblastine 5 mg/m² IV	Day 1, 29 Day 1, 8, 15, 22, 29
Cisplatin/carboplatin and pemetrexed (nonsquamous carcinoma only)[38,39]	Cisplatin 75 mg/m² IV or Carboplatin AUC 5 mg/mL/min IV over 30 min Pemetrexed 500 mg/m² IV	Every 3 wk × 3 cycles (cisplatin) × 4 cycles (carboplatin)

Abbreviation: AUC, area under the plasma concentration time curve.

NSCLC compared 3 radiation treatment groups: low dose (36–45 Gy), standard dose (45–54 Gy), and high dose (54–74 Gy).[42] All patients were also treated with neoadjuvant chemotherapy and underwent surgical resection. In both univariate and multivariate analysis, patients who were treated with standard-dose radiation therapy had longer overall survival (univariate: median 38.3 vs 31.8 and 29.0 months for low-dose and high-dose groups, respectively, $P = .0089$; multivariate: HR 0.77, 95% CI 0.64–0.92 for low-dose group and HR 0.81, 95% CI 0.67–0.98 for high-dose group). Patients treated with high-dose radiation therapy had significantly less residual nodal disease, but this did not translate into a survival advantage. Furthermore, patients treated with the standard therapy dose had fewer prolonged hospitalizations.

Today, the total thoracic radiation doses administered in the preoperative treatment of NSCLC range from 50 to 60 Gy.[7,36–38] It is common to give a total dose of 54 Gy and then evaluate the response. The dose is given in fractions, usually about 1.8 to 2.0 Gy per day for 5 days per week, for a total of 5 to 7 weeks. Fractionation allows noncancerous cells to heal and also allows for cells in a more radioresistant phase of the cell cycle to transition to a more radiosensitive phase for treatment. If the response is insufficient to allow for surgical resection, additional concurrent chemoradiotherapy is given to a higher total dose. Patients are allowed a 4- to 6-week recovery period (as measured from completion of neoadjuvant therapy) before proceeding to surgery (**Table 3**).

Radiation therapy is often combined with preoperative chemotherapy in concurrent or sequential administration. Chemotherapy may induce cell cycle synchronization thereby decreasing the number of cells in the G_0 phase of the cell cycle, which are not as radiosensitive. Sequential administration is usually selected to allow for recovery from side effects before beginning the next therapy.

In patients with locally advanced NSCLC, studies have shown that concurrent neoadjuvant chemotherapy and radiation therapy improves the likelihood of a complete (R0) resection. Fifty-nine percent of the patients with stage IIIA or IIIB NSCLC in the SWOG 8805 study had a partial or complete response to induction chemoradiotherapy.[7] The German Lung Cancer Cooperative Group showed increased mediastinal downstaging and pathologic response with the addition of chemoradiation treatment in patients with stage III NSCLC.[18] In the West Japan Thoracic Oncology Group phase III study (WJTOG9904) comparing patients with stage IIIA(N2) NSCLC treated with neoadjuvant chemotherapy and radiation versus just neoadjuvant chemotherapy, tumor downstaging was 40% versus 21%, respectively.[43] In this same study, the overall survival with and without tumor downstaging was found to be 55.0 and 9.4 months,

Table 3
Thoracic radiotherapy regimens and schedules of administration as matched with their recommended concurrent chemotherapy (see Table 2)

Total Radiotherapy Dose	Concurrent Chemotherapies	Frequency of Administration
61 Gy[7]	Cisplatin and etoposide	7 wk/34 daily fractions
63 Gy[36]	Carboplatin and paclitaxel	7 wk/34 daily fractions
63 Gy[37]	Cisplatin and vinblastine	7 wk/34 daily fractions (1.8 Gy × 25 fractions, then 2.0 Gy × 9 fractions)
70 Gy[38,39]	Cisplatin/carboplatin and pemetrexed (nonsquamous carcinoma only)	7 wk/35 daily fractions

respectively (HR = 3.39, P = .001). Good therapeutic response and improved local disease control increases the likelihood of complete surgical resection.

Finally, a phase II, multi-institutional trial by the Radiation Therapy Oncology Group (0229) assessed the ability of neoadjuvant concurrent chemotherapy and high-dose radiation to increase the rate of mediastinal nodal sterilization in patients with N2/N3 NSCLC as well as the surgical outcomes in this setting[44]. In this study, patients with stage III NSCLC were evaluated by surgical, medical, and radiation oncology. Surgeons were required to demonstrate expertise in surgery after neoadjuvant chemoradiotherapy. All patients underwent pathologic lymph node staging using bronchoscopy and transbronchial needle aspiration, mediastinoscopy, or thoracoscopy before treatment. Induction chemoradiation consisted of carboplatin/paclitaxel and 61.2 Gy to the mediastinum and the primary tumor. The lymph nodes were then reassessed before or at the time of resection. The primary end point of the study was mediastinal nodal clearance. Of 57 eligible patients, 43 (75%) were evaluable for the primary end point, of which 27 had achieved mediastinal nodal clearance. Thirty-seven patients underwent surgical resection; 34 lobectomies and 3 pneumonectomies were performed. Twenty-three of the 37 patients underwent surgery per protocol and 36 of 37 had adequate lymph node sampling. Morbidity and mortality were a 16% (6 of 37) incidence of grade 3 postoperative pulmonary complications and one death, respectively. This study concluded that neoadjuvant concurrent chemoradiotherapy can effectively sterilize known mediastinal nodal disease. Trimodality therapy remains a viable option for carefully selected patients with stage III NSCLC.

DEVELOPING THERAPIES

Targeted therapies, which block mutant proteins or biochemical pathways, are being developed for preoperative treatment of NSCLC. Gefitinib is an epidermal growth factor receptor inhibitor that was found in a phase III trial treating patients with metastatic NSCLC to significantly improve progression-free survival as compared with carboplatin and paclitaxel.[45] However, there was no significant difference found in overall survival.[46] Clinical trials (such as NCT00062270, NCT00188617, and NCT00103051) are underway to evaluate the benefits of preoperatively treating patients with stages I through III NSCLC with gefitinib.

Immunotherapeutics are also being developed and tested as a treatment of NSCLC. Although traditional chemotherapy aims to target rapidly dividing cancer cells, immunotherapy aims to prime the immune system to recognize cancer cells as foreign targets. Most studies evaluating the efficacy of immunotherapies have been for advanced, unresectable NSCLC or for recurrences. The median progression-free survival of patients with advanced NSCLC after treatment with nivolumab, a programmed death 1 inhibitor antibody, was 3.5 months versus 2.8 months with docetaxel (HR 0.62, 95% CI 0.47–0.81, $P<.001$).[47] When ipilimumab, an inhibitor antibody that targets cytotoxic T-lymphocyte-associated protein 4, was combined with paclitaxel and carboplatin and given in phases for treatment of patients with stage IIIB/IV disease, there was improvement in progression-free survival (HR 0.69, P = .02).[48] These studies have shown that antibodies specifically targeting immune system checkpoints or immune cells result in improved survival in advanced NSCLC.

Although there are phase I to III clinical trials evaluating the benefits of immunotherapeutics, few studies have evaluated the effect of these therapies on the surgery itself when used as neoadjuvant treatment. Ratto and colleagues[49] conducted a phase I/II pilot study in which patients with stage IIIA(N2) NSCLC were randomized to receive preoperative immunotherapy in addition to cisplatin and gemcitabine. Their study showed a statistically significant overall survival benefit for patients who received recombinant interleukin 2 and peripheral blood mononuclear cells (tumor-infiltrating lymphocytes). Surgical resection after the addition of preoperative immunotherapy was found to be safe and feasible in their study; but the number of patients in this experimental arm was 13, so further evaluation is warranted. A phase II trial is underway assessing the addition of an immune system checkpoint inhibitor, antiprogrammed death-ligand 1 antibody, to the preoperative and postoperative treatment of patients with stage IIIA(N2) NSCLC (NCT02572843).

EVALUATION AFTER NEOADJUVANT THERAPY

Patients treated with neoadjuvant therapy are allowed a period of 4 to 6 weeks for recovery before surgical resection. During this time, restaging is performed with a PET/CT scan to assess the response to the preoperative therapy. Patients with stable disease or a response to treatment will proceed to surgery. The goal for neoadjuvant therapy is to induce a pathologic complete response or at least decrease the primary tumor size and the mediastinal nodal disease. Patients with advanced disease predicted to be amenable to surgery after preoperative therapy are reimaged 1 to 2 weeks before the completion of therapy. Rebiopsy or repeat mediastinoscopy may be warranted to assess therapy response. If there is evidence of a good response (ie, downstaged disease, decrease in primary tumor size), patients are deemed eligible for surgical resection and finish the predetermined course of neoadjuvant therapy before surgery. If the patients' disease is still unresectable, the chemoradiotherapy course may be altered to a higher, definitive dose or a different chemotherapy is considered followed by further staging before surgery. Using this approach, a minimally invasive or interventional biopsy should be done before treatment if possible, saving a mediastinoscopy for restaging after the completion of treatment. Choosing to offer surgery to patients with no or only minimal residual mediastinal disease will help select the best candidates for surgery and long-term cure.

TREATMENT RESISTANCE/COMPLICATIONS

Although the preferred neoadjuvant treatment regimen includes platinum-based chemotherapy, no clinical trial has established the optimal concurrent chemoradiotherapy regimen. Chemoresistance has been documented with all chemotherapeutics[50] in an adjuvant or definitive therapy setting and is often treated by changing to a different course of drugs. There are also agents that may help restore the function of the chemotherapy[51] and new chemotherapies being developed to treat NSCLC refractory to the currently available drugs.[52] Although chemoresistance is monitored when chemotherapies are given for adjuvant or definitive treatment, studies are developing methods of assessing biomarker response levels as a means of evaluating neoadjuvant response.[53,54]

Neoadjuvant therapy has associated toxicities. Side effects from neoadjuvant therapy include radiation pneumonitis, nausea, vomiting, fatigue, pain, blood disorders, and drug-specific effects. The objective of preoperative therapy is to derive the most benefit from the regimen while minimizing the side effects. To achieve this goal, the clinical team continuously reviews patients' tolerance of the treatment regimen, encourages patients to report all side effects, and provides supportive treatment of the side effects when possible. Concurrent chemoradiotherapy may be changed to a sequential regimen to help patients tolerate the treatments.

Surgery after neoadjuvant therapy is also associated with complications, such as limitations to the extent of resection. In the GLCCG study, 35% of the patients in the intervention group (with preoperative radiation) and 35% of the patients in the control group (with postoperative radiation) underwent a pneumonectomy.[18] The treatment-related mortality was increased for those who had preoperative radiation therapy (14% vs 6%), and the treatment-related mortality was also increased for those who had preoperative radiation undergoing a lobectomy or bilobectomy (8% vs 2%); but these differences were not found to be statistically significant. However, the investigators caution against performing a pneumonectomy in patients with stage III NSCLC after treatment with induction chemoradiotherapy because of the higher mortality risk found in the study.

Many other studies have also found an association between pneumonectomy and increased operative mortality in a multimodality treatment setting (both neoadjuvant and adjuvant).[7,10,55,56] In a retrospective review of 315 patients with NSCLC who underwent pneumonectomy, d'Amato and colleagues[55] compared the outcomes of patients who had induction therapy versus those who had surgery alone. Sixty-eight patients underwent induction chemotherapy (mostly platinum-based regimens), and 33 of the 68 also had neoadjuvant radiation (average dose 45.6 Gy), whereas 247 had surgery alone. The clinical characteristics between the patient cohorts were well matched. The overall operative mortality was 29 of 315, with 21 deaths after right pneumonectomy versus 8 deaths after left pneumonectomy. Thirty-day mortality was 21.0% in the induction therapy group versus 6.1% in the surgery only group (odds ratio 4.01, 95% CI 1.826–8.804, $P = .0007$). When postoperative complications (bronchopleural fistula, respiratory failure, pneumonia, arrhythmia) were evaluated, no significant differences were noted between the two groups. Interestingly, when the entire cohort of 315 was evaluated, age was found to be predictive of operative mortality in 13 of 86 patients greater than 70 years old, compared with 16 of 229 patients less than 70 years old (HR 1.77, $P = .046$).

European studies have reported no increased association between operative mortality and pneumonectomy in the setting of multimodality therapy.[57,58] To date, no prospective, randomized clinical trial has been conducted to clarify the association between operative mortality and pneumonectomy after induction therapy. A study from Korea reviewing 186 patients undergoing surgical resection after neoadjuvant chemoradiation for stage IIIA(N2) NSCLC found that the 30-day mortality rate was higher for bilobectomy as well as pneumonectomy (8.7%, 7.1%) as compared with that for lobectomy (1.5%).[59] Caution should be exercised in considering an extent of resection greater than a lobectomy when treating patients with surgery, chemotherapy, and radiation therapy.

OUTCOMES AND LONG-TERM RECOMMENDATIONS

After completion of therapy, the patients' treatment response is evaluated. The pathologic stage of the resected specimen along with prognostic genetic markers are used to assess the need for adjuvant therapy. If no further therapy is warranted (or when adjuvant therapy has been completed), follow-up is initiated. The ACCP has recommended the following for follow-up of patients treated for lung cancer[44,60]:

1. After curative intent therapy, regular follow-up intervals should be scheduled with surveillance to detect new disease or recurrence in the first 3 to 6 months.
2. For patients with no new evidence of disease, further follow-up with imaging is recommended at 6-month intervals for the first 2 years after treatment. The follow-up interval may be increased to annually after 2 years, and all patients should be trained to report suspicious symptoms that may indicate recurrence/new disease.

3. If possible, the original physician who diagnosed the primary cancer with the multi-disciplinary team should remain as the primary clinician and team.
4. After curative intent therapy, blood tests, tumor markers, sputum cytology, PET scanning, and fluorescence bronchoscopy are not recommended for surveillance.
5. Patients are strongly encouraged to refrain from using tobacco products and are offered pharmacologic and behavioral therapy to assist with cessation.

SUMMARY/DISCUSSION

Patients presenting with a new lung tumor should undergo a thorough staging assessment. This assessment includes obtaining a pathologic diagnosis of the primary tumor and the mediastinal lymph node disease if there is suspicion for metastasis in this location. Neoadjuvant chemotherapy, with a platinum-based drug regimen, alone or with concurrent radiotherapy is recommended for resectable stage IIIA(N2) NSCLC. Preoperative chemotherapy is given to treat micrometastatic disease, and preoperative radiation therapy is given to increase the likelihood of decreasing the primary tumor size and achieving a complete resection. Many clinical trials are currently underway, testing new drugs and drug combinations to find the regimen with the best prognostic effect. Future studies may develop biomarker assays to be applied to preoperative biopsies to help determine the most effective neoadjuvant regimen for a given patient diagnosed with NSCLC.

REFERENCES

1. World Health Organization, Media Centre. Cancer. 2015. Available at: http://www.who.int/mediacentre/factsheets/fs297/en/. Accessed October 7, 2015.
2. Chansky K, Sculier JP, Crowley JJ, et al, International Staging Committee and Participating Institutions. The International Association for the Study of Lung Cancer Staging Project: prognostic factors and pathologic TNM stage in surgically managed non-small cell lung cancer. J Thorac Oncol 2009;4:792–801.
3. Goldstraw P, Crowley J, Chansky K, et al, International Association for the Study of Lung Cancer International Staging Committee, Participating Institutions. The IASLC lung cancer staging project: proposals for the revision of the TNM stage groupings in the forthcoming (seventh) edition of the TNM Classification of malignant tumors. J Thorac Oncol 2007;2:706–14.
4. Sugarbaker DJ, Herndon J, Kohman LJ, et al. Results of cancer and leukemia group B protocol 8935. A multiinstitutional phase II trimodality trial for stage IIIA (N2) non-small-cell lung cancer. Cancer and Leukemia Group B Thoracic Surgery Group. J Thorac Cardiovasc Surg 1995;109:483–5.
5. Strauss GM, Herndon JE, Sherman DD, et al. Neoadjuvant chemotherapy and radiotherapy followed by surgery in stage IIIA non-small-cell carcinoma of the lung: report of a Cancer and Leukemia Group B phase II study. J Clin Oncol 1992;10:1237–44.
6. Jaklitsch MT, Herndon JE, DeCamp MM, et al. Nodal downstaging predicts survival following induction chemotherapy for stage IIIA (N2) non-small cell lung cancer in CALGB protocol #8935. J Surg Oncol 2006;94:599–606.
7. Albain KS, Rusch VW, Crowley JJ, et al. Concurrent cisplatin/etoposide plus chest radiotherapy followed by surgery for stages IIIA (N2) and IIIB non-small-cell lung cancer: mature results of Southwest Oncology Group phase II study 8805. J Clin Oncol 1995;13:1880–92.

8. Rosell R, Gomez-Codina J, Camps C, et al. A randomized trial comparing preoperative chemotherapy plus surgery with surgery alone in patients with non-small-cell lung cancer. N Engl J Med 1994;330:153–8.

9. Roth JA, Fossella F, Komaki R, et al. A randomized trial comparing perioperative chemotherapy and surgery with surgery alone in resectable stage IIIA non-small-cell lung cancer. J Natl Cancer Inst 1994;86:673–80.

10. Bueno R, Richards WG, Swanson SJ, et al. Nodal stage after induction therapy for stage IIIA lung cancer determines patient survival. Ann Thorac Surg 2000; 70:1826–31.

11. Pisters KM, Vallieres E, Crowley JJ, et al. Surgery with or without preoperative paclitaxel and carboplatin in early-stage non-small-cell lung cancer: Southwest Oncology Group Trial S9900, an intergroup, randomized, phase III trial. J Clin Oncol 2010;28:1843–949.

12. Endo C, Saito Y, Iwanami H, et al, North-east Japan Study Group for Lung Cancer Surgery. A randomized trial of postoperative UFT therapy in p stage I, II non-small cell lung cancer: North-east Japan Study Group for Lung Cancer Surgery. Lung Cancer 2003;40:181–6.

13. Arriagada R, Bergman B, Dunant A, et al, International Adjuvant Lung Cancer Trial Collaborative Group. Cisplatin-based adjuvant chemotherapy in patients with completely resected non-small-cell lung cancer. N Engl J Med 2004;350: 351–60.

14. Winton T, Livingston R, Johnson D, et al. Vinorelbine plus cisplatin vs. observation in resected non-small-cell lung cancer. N Engl J Med 2005;352:2589–97.

15. Strauss GM, Herndon JE 2nd, Maddaus MA, et al. Adjuvant paclitaxel plus carboplatin compared with observation in stage IB non-small-cell lung cancer: CALGB 9633 with the Cancer and Leukemia Group B, Radiation Therapy Oncology Group, and North Central Cancer Treatment Group Study Groups. J Clin Oncol 2008;26:5043–51.

16. Felip E, Rosell R, Maestre JA, et al. Preoperative chemotherapy plus surgery versus surgery plus adjuvant chemotherapy versus surgery alone in early-stage non-small-cell lung cancer. J Clin Oncol 2010;28:3138–45.

17. NSCLC Meta-analysis Collaborative Group. Preoperative chemotherapy for non-small-cell lung cancer: a systematic review and meta-analysis of individual participant data. Lancet 2014;383:1561–71.

18. Thomas M, Rube C, Hoffknecht P, et al, German Lung Cancer Cooperative Group. Effect of preoperative chemoradiation in addition to preoperative chemotherapy: a randomised trial in stage III non-small-cell lung cancer. Lancet Oncol 2008;9:636–48.

19. Bueno R, Hughes E, Wagner S, et al. Validation of a molecular and pathological model for five-year mortality risk in patients with early stage lung adenocarcinoma. J Thorac Oncol 2015;10:67–73.

20. Wang EH, Corso CD, Rutter CE, et al. Postoperative radiation therapy is associated with improved overall survival in incompletely resected stage II and III non-small-cell lung cancer. J Clin Oncol 2015;33:2727–34.

21. Stupp R, Mayer M, Kann R, et al. Neoadjuvant chemotherapy and radiotherapy followed by surgery in selected patients with stage IIIB non-small-cell lung cancer: a multicentre phase II trial. Lancet Oncol 2009;10:785–93.

22. Edge SB, Byrd DR, Compton CC, et al. AJCC cancer staging handbook. New York: Springer; 2009.

23. Ettinger DS, Wood DE, Akerley W, et al. Non-small cell lung cancer, version 1.2015. J Natl Compr Canc Netw 2014;12:1738–61.

24. Robinson LA, Ruckdeschel JC, Wagner H Jr, et al, American College of Chest Physicians. Treatment of non-small cell lung cancer-stage IIIA: ACCP evidence-based clinical practice guidelines (2nd edition). Chest 2007;132:243S–65S.
25. Jaklitsch MT, Strauss GM, Sugarbaker DJ. Neoadjuvant and adjuvant therapy in the management of locally advanced non-small-cell lung cancer. World J Surg 1993;17:729–34.
26. Ettinger DS, Akerley W, Bepler G, et al. Non-small cell lung cancer. J Natl Compr Canc Netw 2010;8:740–801.
27. Andre F, Grunenwald D, Pignon JP, et al. Survival of patients with resected N2 non-small-cell lung cancer: evidence for a subclassification and implications. J Clin Oncol 2000;18:2981–9.
28. Rusch VW, Giroux DJ, Kraut MJ, et al. Induction chemoradiation and surgical resection for superior sulcus non-small-cell lung carcinomas: long-term results of Southwest Oncology Group Trial 9416 (Intergroup Trial 0160). J Clin Oncol 2007;25:313–8.
29. Patterson GA, Piazza D, Pearson FG, et al. Significance of metastatic disease in subaortic lymph nodes. Ann Thorac Surg 1987;43:155–9.
30. Oken MM, Creech RH, Tormey DC, et al. Toxicity and response criteria of the Eastern Cooperative Oncology Group. Am J Clin Oncol 1982;5:649–55.
31. Buccheri G, Ferrigno D, Tamburini M. Karnofsky and ECOG performance status scoring in lung cancer: a prospective, longitudinal study of 536 patients from a single institution. Eur J Cancer 1996;32A:1135–41.
32. Firat S, Bousamra M, Gore E, et al. Comorbidity and KPS are independent prognostic factors in stage I non-small-cell lung cancer. Int J Radiat Oncol Biol Phys 2002;52:1047–57.
33. Kocher F, Pircher A, Mohn-Staudner A, et al. Multicenter phase II study evaluating docetaxel and cisplatin as neoadjuvant induction regimen prior to surgery or radiochemotherapy with docetaxel, followed by adjuvant docetaxel therapy in chemonaive patients with NSCLC stage II, IIIA, IIIB (TAX-AT 1.203 Trial). Lung Cancer 2014;85:395–400.
34. Peterson P, Park K, Fossella F, et al. Is pemetrexed more effective in adenocarcinoma and large cell lung cancer than in squamous cell carcinoma? A retrospective analysis of a phase III trial of pemetrexed vs docetaxel in previously treated patients with advanced non-small cell lung cancer (NSCLC): P2–328. J Thorac Oncol 2007;8:S851.
35. Scagliotti G, Hanna N, Fossella F, et al. The differential efficacy of pemetrexed according to NSCLC histology: a review of two phase III studies. Oncologist 2009; 14:253–63.
36. Belani CP, Choy H, Bonomi P, et al. Combined chemoradiotherapy regimens of paclitaxel and carboplatin for locally advanced non-small-cell lung cancer: a randomized phase II locally advanced multi-modality protocol. J Clin Oncol 2005;23: 5883–91.
37. Curran WJ Jr, Paulus R, Langer CJ, et al. Sequential vs. concurrent chemoradiation for stage III non-small cell lung cancer: randomized phase III trial RTOG 9410. J Natl Cancer Inst 2011;103:1452–60.
38. Govindan R, Bogart J, Stinchcombe T, et al. Randomized phase II study of pemetrexed, carboplatin, and thoracic radiation with or without cetuximab in patients with locally advanced unresectable non-small-cell lung cancer: Cancer and Leukemia Group B trial 30407. J Clin Oncol 2011;29:3120–5.
39. Schuette WH, Groschel A, Sebastian M, et al. A randomized phase II study of pemetrexed in combination with cisplatin or carboplatin as first-line therapy for

patients with locally advanced or metastatic non-small-cell lung cancer. Clin Lung Cancer 2013;14:215–23.

40. Perez CA, Stanley K, Rubin P, et al. A prospective randomized study of various irradiation doses and fractionation schedules in the treatment of inoperable non-oat-cell carcinoma of the lung. Preliminary report by the Radiation Therapy Oncology Group. Cancer 1980;45:44–53.

41. Cerfolio RJ, Bryant AS, Spencer SA, et al. Pulmonary resection after high-dose and low-dose chest irradiation. Ann Thorac Surg 2005;80:1224–30.

42. Sher DJ, Fidler MJ, Seder CW, et al. Relationship between radiation therapy dose and outcome in patients treated with neoadjuvant chemoradiation therapy and surgery for stage IIIA non-small cell lung cancer: a population-based, comparative effectiveness analysis. Int J Radiat Oncol Biol Phys 2015;92:307–16.

43. Katakami N, Tada H, Mitsudomi T, et al. A phase 3 study of induction treatment with concurrent chemoradiotherapy versus chemotherapy before surgery in patients with pathologically confirmed N2 stage IIIA nonsmall cell lung cancer (WJTOG9903). Cancer 2012;118:126–35.

44. Suntharalingam M, Paulus R, Edelman MJ, et al. Radiation Therapy Oncology Group Protocol 02-29: a phase II trial of neoadjuvant therapy with concurrent chemotherapy and full-dose radiation therapy followed by surgical resection and consolidative therapy for locally advanced non-small cell carcinoma of the lung. Int J Radiat Oncol Biol Phys 2012;84(2):456–63.

45. Maemondo M, Inoue A, Kobayashi K, et al. Gefitinib or chemotherapy for non-small-cell lung cancer with mutated EGFR. N Engl J Med 2010;362:2380–8.

46. Inoue A, Kobayashi K, Maemondo M, et al. Updated overall survival results from a randomized phase III trial comparing gefitinib with carboplatin-paclitaxel for chemo-naive non-small cell lung cancer with sensitive EGFR gene mutations (NEJ002). Ann Oncol 2013;24:54–9.

47. Brahmer J, Reckamp KL, Baas P, et al. Nivolumab versus docetaxel in advanced squamous-cell non-small-cell lung cancer. N Engl J Med 2015;373:123–35.

48. Lynch TJ, Bondarenko I, Luft A, et al. Ipilimumab in combination with paclitaxel and carboplatin as first-line treatment in stage IIIB/IV non-small-cell lung cancer: results from a randomized, double-blind, multicenter phase II study. J Clin Oncol 2012;30:2046–54.

49. Ratto GB, Costa R, Maineri P, et al. Neo-adjuvant chemo/immunotherapy in the treatment of stage III (N2) non-small cell lung cancer: a phase I/II pilot study. Int J Immunopathol Pharmacol 2011;24:1005–16.

50. D'Amato T, Landreneau R, McKenna R, et al. Prevalence of in vitro extreme chemotherapy resistance in resected non small-cell lung cancer. Ann Thorac Surg 2006;81:440–6.

51. Sequist LV, Fidias PM, Temel JS, et al. Phase 1-2a multicenter dose-ranging study of canfosfamide in combination with carboplatin and paclitaxel as first-line therapy for patients with advanced non-small cell lung cancer. J Thorac Oncol 2009;4:1389–96.

52. Mauer AM, Cohen EE, Ma PC, et al. A phase II study of ABT-751 in patients with advanced non-small cell lung cancer. J Thorac Oncol 2008;3:631–6.

53. Rocco G. The surgeon's role in molecular biology. J Thorac Cardiovasc Surg 2012;144:S18–22.

54. Meert AP, Martin B, Verdebout JM, et al. Correlation of different markers (p53, EGF-R, c-erbB-2, Ki-67) expression in the diagnostic biopsies and the corresponding resected tumors in non-small cell lung cancer. Lung Cancer 2004;44: 295–301.

55. d'Amato TA, Ashrafi AS, Schuchert MJ, et al. Risk of pneumonectomy after induction therapy for locally advanced non-small cell lung cancer. Ann Thorac Surg 2009;88:1079–85.

56. Albain KS, Swann RS, Rusch VW, et al. Radiotherapy plus chemotherapy with or without surgical resection for stage III non-small-cell lung cancer: a phase III randomised controlled trial. Lancet 2009;374:379–86.

57. Mansour Z, Kochetkova EA, Ducrocq X, et al. Induction chemotherapy does not increase the operative risk of pneumonectomy! Eur J Cardiothorac Surg 2007;31:181–5.

58. Gudbjartsson T, Gyllstedt E, Pikwer A, et al. Early surgical results after pneumonectomy for non-small cell lung cancer are not affected by preoperative radiotherapy and chemotherapy. Ann Thorac Surg 2008;86:376–82.

59. Cho JH, Kim J, Kim K, et al. Risk associated with bilobectomy after neoadjuvant concurrent chemoradiotherapy for stage IIIA/N2 non-small-cell lung cancer. World J Surg 2012;36:1199–205.

60. Rubins J, Unger M, Colice GL, American College of Chest Physicians. Follow-up and surveillance of the lung cancer patient following curative intent therapy: ACCP evidence-based clinical practice (2nd edition). Chest 2007;132:355S–67S.

Adjuvant Therapy for Stage I and II Non–Small Cell Lung Cancer

Evan C. Naylor, MD

KEYWORDS

- Adjuvant • Chemotherapy • Non–small cell lung cancer

KEY POINTS

- Adjuvant chemotherapy administered after complete surgical resection of non–small cell lung cancer results in an absolute survival benefit at 5 years of approximately 5%.
- Patient factors, such as comorbidities, life expectancy, and performance status, and tumor characteristics, such as histology, size, surgical margins, and nodal involvement, must be considered when selecting appropriate patients for chemotherapy.
- Cisplatin-based combination chemotherapy remains the standard of care for optimizing outcomes in patients with higher risk stage I to stage III non–small cell lung cancer.

INTRODUCTION

Patients with surgically resected early-stage non–small cell lung cancer (NSCLC) have a relatively high risk of distant recurrence and death despite optimal surgical outcomes. In the United States, patients with localized disease have a 54.8% 5-year overall survival, whereas those with regional nodal disease have a 27.4% 5-year overall survival.[1]

Administration of systemic cytotoxic chemotherapy to patients with no known residual disease in the postoperative period had been unsuccessful in early clinical trials using single-agent alkylating agents. In 2004 and 2005, 2 trials demonstrated a benefit in survival in a subset of these patients,[2,3] and further trials and meta-analyses have supported this finding. Identification of patients who derive the most significant improvement from chemotherapy in this setting has required numerous international clinical trials and the pooling of individual patient data into large meta-analyses.

PATIENT EVALUATION OVERVIEW

When evaluating patients for adjuvant therapy, the oncologist and the patient must weigh the overall benefit of therapy in long-term survival against the risk of complications. Several patient and tumor characteristics require thorough assessment.

Disclosure Statement: The author has nothing to disclose.
Hematology and Oncology, Meridian Cancer Care, Southern Ocean Medical Center, 1140 Route 72 West, Manahawkin, NJ 08050, USA
E-mail address: enaylor@meridianhealth.com

Surg Oncol Clin N Am 25 (2016) 585–599
http://dx.doi.org/10.1016/j.soc.2016.03.003
surgonc.theclinics.com

Tumor Factors

TNM stage

The features of the resected tumor most critical to that determination are the size of the primary tumor, lymph node involvement, grade of the tumor, and histology. Each of these plays a part in the risk of developing recurrent disease and choice of adjuvant therapy. In patients with negative regional lymph nodes, increasing tumor size and T stage have been shown to be associated with a decrease in long-term survival.[4]

The appropriate use of chemotherapy in patients with negative lymph nodes has been a matter of much debate. Many experts recommend administering adjuvant chemotherapy in patients with a primary tumor greater than or equal to 4 cm based on a survival benefit seen in cancer and leukemia group B (CALGB) 9633.[5] Several retrospective studies suggest there may be a benefit in patients with tumors greater than 2 cm, however.[6] This benefit has not been seen in prospective trials.

Tumor grade and lymphatic/vascular invasion

Higher tumor grade and the presence of lymphatic or vascular invasion may be associated with increased risk of recurrence,[7,8] and retrospective data indicate that some benefit may exist in treating such patients with chemotherapy.[9]

Histology

NSCLC consists of several different subtypes. Studies of patients with metastatic lung cancer have demonstrated that certain histologic subtypes are more likely to respond to a particular agent. The 2 most common histologies in NSCLC, adenocarcinoma and squamous cell carcinoma, have similar rates of disease recurrence.[10] Patients with metastatic adenocarcinoma seem to benefit from platinum-based doublets using pemetrexed (Alimta), whereas patients with metastatic squamous cell carcinoma benefit more from doublets incorporating gemcitabine (Gemzar).[11,12] Whether such benefits remain relevant in the adjuvant setting is unclear.

The new International Association for the Study of Lung Cancer/American Thoracic Society/European Respiratory Society classification system further divides adenocarcinoma into histologic patterns. Patients with solid- and micropapillary-predominant lung adenocarcinoma have the poorest prognosis,[13–17] and these subtypes appear to derive a disease-free survival benefit from adjuvant chemotherapy.[18] Some evidence suggests that lepidic-, acinar-, and papillary-predominant tumors do not show a significant benefit with the addition of adjuvant chemotherapy.

Margin status

The role of adjuvant chemotherapy in patients with positive margins of resection was evaluated in a National Cancer Database review.[19] The investigators found an improvement in 5-year mortality (adjusted hazard ratio 0.75) in patients receiving adjuvant chemotherapy in this setting, regardless of tumor size.

Single biomarkers

The current staging system based on tumor size and pattern of dissemination is inadequate in predicting the expected outcome for individual patients with cancer. A treatment plan that is personalized to identify those deriving the most benefit from adjuvant therapy would be useful to provide justification for or against chemotherapy in the context of the expected complications and risks involved for patients. Recent studies have sought to identify the prognostic and predictive factors related to the genomic characteristics of a tumor that could affect adjuvant and neoadjuvant treatment choices for NSCLC.

The absence or presence of a biomarker can assist in determining the probability of success in adjuvant chemotherapy for patients with cancer. A substudy of the International Adjuvant Lung Cancer (IALT) trial examined Excision repair cross-complementation group 1 (ERCC1) expression in tumor cells.[20] The results indicated that patients who had ERCC1-negative tumors had a longer survival when receiving cisplatin (Platinol)-based chemotherapy versus observation. Patients treated with chemotherapy who displayed ERCC1 expression did not have an advantage. Unfortunately, the reliability of ERCC1 immunohistochemical staining has not been consistent when put into large-scale prospective testing.[21]

NRF2 pathway alterations have been shown to activate the oxidative response pathways in tumors.[22] Using tumor tissue from the JBR.10 trial, patients with a gene expression signature of NRF2 pathway activation, but not those with NRF2 pathway-activating somatic alterations, were found to have a benefit from adjuvant cisplatin and vinorelbine (Navelbine).[23]

Furthermore, p53 and RAS are imperative to cell-cycle regulation, apoptosis, transcription, response to stress, and DNA repair. Patients whose tumors demonstrate p53 protein overexpression, compared with those with low expression, have a shorter survival and appear to benefit from adjuvant chemotherapy.[24] p53 and RAS mutations, however, have not shown utility as a predictive biomarker.[24–26]

Prognostic signatures and cell-cycle progression biomarkers

As stated elsewhere, the benefit of adjuvant chemotherapy in patients with stage IB NSCLC is uncertain. Efforts to analyze the risk of disease recurrence based on a single gene in lung cancer have largely been disappointing. Multigene panels have proven useful in similar situations in patients with breast cancer,[27] and to a lesser degree in colon[28] and prostate cancer.[29] Similar investigations in lung cancer are in the early testing stage with promising results, although not yet widely accepted.

Microarray profiling of tumors in JBR.10 revealed a 15-gene signature capable of providing prognostic and predictive information.[30] This signature was retrospectively validated in a set of patients including a number with stage IB disease. Prognosis was also accurately predicted in a separate prospective study of patients with stage I disease.[31] A benefit for adjuvant chemotherapy with cisplatin and vinorelbine was seen only in patients with disease characterized by this signature as high risk.

A messenger RNA expression signature of cell-cycle progression (CCP) genes was evaluated by Wistuba and colleagues[32] and was found to be a strong independent predictor of survival in patients with stage I and II lung cancer. Although the CCP score may be useful in determining prognosis and selecting patients at the highest risk of distant recurrence, studies supporting its use as a predictive marker are lacking.

Host Factors

Age

The average age of diagnosis of lung cancer is 70, and 36.7% of patients are 75 years old or older.[1] In elderly patients, chemotherapy is often perceived as carrying an increased risk of morbidity and perhaps mortality. As a result, patients with lung cancer and their physicians often reach the decision not to pursue guideline-based therapies for various reasons.[33] Cisplatin, in particular, may lead to acute and chronic kidney injury, long-term auditory symptoms, and peripheral neuropathy, which are expected to lead to a decreased quality of life. Declines in renal function are not universal in the elderly, however.[34] For some older patients, risking a decline in functional status due to peripheral neuropathy and gait instability or hearing loss does not justify a miniscule improvement in overall survival.

Life expectancy often impacts decisions on adjuvant therapy. For example, a patient unlikely to survive beyond 5 years due to age or comorbidities, such as chronic obstructive pulmonary disease or cardiac disease, would be expected to derive fewer life-years saved from intensive chemotherapy than a younger and healthier patient.

The benefit of adjuvant chemotherapy in an elderly population has been explored in several studies and substudies. The Lung Adjuvant Cisplatin Analysis (LACE) pooled analysis of 5 adjuvant trials explored the role of age on benefit and toxicity with chemotherapy.[35] Notably, only 9% of patients in this analysis were age 70 or beyond, and only 1.3% of patients were older than 75, relatively small numbers compared with those seen in clinical practice in our aging population. This analysis demonstrated that elderly patients more often had initial dose reductions of cisplatin, and that fewer than 60% were able to complete more than half of the planned adjuvant cycles. Patients age 70 or older did not experience an increase in specific or overall toxicity, or in treatment-related death. Whether this surprising outcome is due to more frequent dose reductions or dose omissions in this group is unknown.

The JBR.10 study looked at treatment outcomes in elderly patients, defined as those more than 65 years old.[36] The chemotherapy benefit in elderly patients was similar to that seen in younger patients. Only 23 patients in the study were older than 75 years, however, creating some difficulty in generalizing these results to this population. Toxicity was similar between the young and elderly age groups, although elderly patients received fewer doses of chemotherapy and lower dose intensity. They were also noted to discontinue chemotherapy more often due to refusal.

A recent Surveillance, Epidemiology, and End Results (SEER)-Medicare database analysis evaluated the use of adjuvant chemotherapy in patients older than 65 years of age with T1-2 N1 NSCLC between 1992 and 2006.[37] Chemotherapy was administered to 28.2% of eligible patients. Five-year overall survival was 35.8% in those receiving chemotherapy compared with 28.0% of those not receiving it. The study was limited in that the patients receiving chemotherapy were generally younger and more had received radiation therapy. Other population-based data[38,39] and the recent Cochrane meta-analysis[40] have shown similar benefits in older patients, although those older than the age of 75 or 80 receiving chemotherapy were not well represented.

Comorbidity and performance status
Comorbid conditions have been shown to impact survival in both early- and late-stage NSCLC.[41] In patients with stage I lung cancer, Karnofsky performance score and the presence of comorbidities independently affected long-term outcomes.[42]

The LACE meta-analysis explored the role of Eastern Cooperative Oncology Group (ECOG) performance status (PS) in patients enrolled in its reviewed trials.[43] Improving PS correlated with an increased benefit of adjuvant chemotherapy. In addition, patients with ECOG PS 2 had a suggestion of a detrimental effect from receipt of chemotherapy. Based on this study and similar findings in the Cochrane meta-analysis,[40] adjuvant chemotherapy cannot be routinely recommended in patients with ECOG PS 2 or greater.

Smoking status
Smoking status also has clear implications on recurrence and survival outcomes in postsurgical patients with early-stage lung cancer.[44] In addition, nicotine modulates mitochondrial signaling, thereby inhibiting chemotherapy-induced apoptosis[45] and possibly rendering chemotherapy less effective. To optimize outcomes, current smokers should be counseled on the importance of tobacco cessation.[41,46,47]

Time to adjuvant chemotherapy

The importance of the amount of time between surgery and delivery of adjuvant chemotherapy has been reviewed. A large Canadian series revealed that one-third of patients had a delay of at least 10 weeks, but increased time to surgery did not have an effect on survival.[48] Another recent study of stage II patients receiving adjuvant chemotherapy suggested that time from surgery to delivery of chemotherapy did not influence outcomes, but that the amount of platinum received was a significant factor.[49]

PHARMACOLOGIC TREATMENT OPTIONS

Adjuvant chemotherapy has been evaluated in a series of studies to determine the appropriate patient population and regimen. Combination cisplatin-based chemotherapy has been the most common approach. Individual trials have yielded markedly different results using a wide range of drugs, complicating decisions on chemotherapy for years (**Table 1**).

Cisplatin-based Adjuvant Chemotherapy

Several individual studies have highlighted the importance of chemotherapy. The IALT study consisted of cisplatin-based adjuvant chemotherapy for stages I to III lung cancer.[2] Different doses of cisplatin were prescribed with either vindesine (Eldesine), vinblastine (Velban), vinorelbine, or etoposide (Etopophos; Toposar) after complete resection. Patients receiving treatment demonstrated an improvement in overall

Table 1
Various individual trials of adjuvant chemotherapy

Name of Trial	Stages of NSCLC Involved	Chemotherapy Used	Benefit
ALPI (n = 1209)[52]	Stages I, II, and IIIA	Cisplatin 100 mg/m^2 on day 1 Mitomycin C 8 mg/m^2 on day 1 Vindesine 3 mg/m^2 on day 1 and 8 (every 3 wk for 3 cycles)	5-y OS benefit 1% (NSS) 5-y PFS benefit 4% (NSS)
ANITA (n = 840)[51]	Stages IB–IIIA	Cisplatin 100 mg/m^2 day 1 Vinorelbine 30 mg/m^2 day 1, 8, 15, and 22 (every 4 wk for 4 cycles)	5-y OS benefit 8.6% 7-y OS benefit 8.4%
Big Lung Trial (n = 381)[53]	Stages I–IIIA	Cisplatin 50–80 mg/m^2 Vindesine, vinorelbine, mitomycin/ vinblastine, or mitomycin/ ifosfamide (every 3 wk for 3 cycles)	2-y PFS benefit 2% (NSS) 2-y OS benefit not seen
CALGB 9633 (n = 344)[83]	Stage IB	Carboplatin AUC 6 Paclitaxel 200 mg/m^2 (every 3 wk for 4 cycles)	8-y OS benefit 7% (NSS)
IALT (n = 1867)[2]	Stages I–III	Cisplatin 80–120 mg/m^2 Vindesine, vinblastine, vinorelbine, or etoposide (every 3–4 wk for 3–4 cycles)	5-y OS benefit 4.1% 5-y DFS benefit 5.1%
JBR.10 (n = 482)[3,50]	Stages IB, II	Cisplatin 50 mg/m^2 days 1 and 8 Vinorelbine 25 mg/m^2 days 1, 8, 15, and 22 (every 28 d for 4 cycles)	5-y OS benefit 11%

Abbreviations: AUC, area under the curve; DFS, disease-free survival; NSS, not statistically significant; OS, overall survival; PFS, progression-free survival.

survival of 4.1%. JBR.10 analyzed the overall survival rate of patients as well as the receipt of postoperative adjuvant chemotherapy for stage IB and II NSCLC with cisplatin and vinorelbine.[50] Those receiving adjuvant therapy experienced a greater overall survival, although this benefit appeared to be confined to those with nodal involvement. The Adjuvant Navelbine International Trialist Association (ANITA) trial called for administration of cisplatin and vinorelbine to individuals diagnosed with stage IB to IIIA lung cancer[51] and was consistent with a clinically and statistically significant improvement in overall and progression-free survival.

A few other studies were unable to demonstrate any significant benefit. The Adjuvant Lung Project Italy (ALPI) study treated patients with stages I to IIIA NSCLC with mitomycin (Mutamycin), vindesine, and cisplatin.[52] These results revealed a small and not statistically significant improvement in survival, partly due to low compliance with chemotherapy. The Big Lung Trial enrolled a greater number of patients who were administered various chemotherapy regimens.[53] This study included individuals with stage I to III NSCLC and used various cisplatin-based combination chemotherapy regimens. No survival improvement was identified.

In the absence of clear and consistent signals from the numerous individual adjuvant trials, the LACE and Cochrane meta-analyses pooled patient data across several trials to confirm the overall benefit of adjuvant chemotherapy (**Table 2**). The LACE meta-analysis was undertaken to assess the efficacy and toxicity of adjuvant chemotherapy and included stages I, II, and III.[35] The results verified that adjuvant chemotherapy improves overall and progression-free survival in patients with stages II and III NSCLC. The power of LACE was insufficient to detect an improvement in survival in stage IB NSCLC.

The Cochrane Lung Cancer Group evaluated individual patient data across 26 randomized trials with patients not receiving radiotherapy (n = 8447) and 12 trials using radiotherapy (n = 2660) to determine the effect of adjuvant chemotherapy.[40] A 5-year overall survival benefit was noted with the addition of chemotherapy, with similar results with (64% vs 60%) or without (33% vs 29%) radiotherapy. No clear difference was detected in subgroups based on age, gender, histology, PS, or stage. Moreover, no chemotherapy agents appeared to be superior to any other. In patients undergoing radiotherapy, the timing of treatment with respect to chemotherapy (sequential vs concurrent) did not have an effect on mortality.

A combination of cisplatin and pemetrexed as adjuvant therapy was evaluated in the phase II TREAT study, primarily because of the tolerability and efficacy of this combination in the advanced lung cancer setting.[11] In the TREAT trial, this combination was better tolerated and resulted in more cisplatin administered than cisplatin and vinorelbine.[54] Data on comparative efficacy have not been published, but cisplatin and

Table 2
Meta-analyses of adjuvant chemotherapy trials

Name of Trials	Stages of NSCLC	Number of Patients	Individual Trials	5-y Survival Benefit
LACE[43]	I–III	n = 4584 (radiotherapy planned in 1439)	JBR.10, ALPI, ANITA, IALT, BLT	OS 5.4%; DFS 5.8%
Cochrane Lung Cancer Group[40]	I–III	No radiotherapy; n = 8447 Radiotherapy; n = 2660	26 trials, including above	OS 4.0%

Abbreviations: DFS, disease-free survival; OS, overall survival.

pemetrexed are considered a reasonable option in patients with nonsquamous NSCLC.

A Bayesian analysis of the IALT, JBR.10, and ANITA trials revealed a high likelihood of benefit from cisplatin-based adjuvant chemotherapy.[55] The probability of at least a 4% improvement in 5-year overall survival was estimated at 82%. The actual 5-year overall survival difference in favor of adjuvant chemotherapy was calculated to be as high as, but not likely to exceed, 7%.

Carboplatin-based Adjuvant Chemotherapy

Cisplatin is the preferred platinum compound as the backbone of an adjuvant chemotherapy regimen, based primarily on studies suggesting superiority of the drug in advanced lung cancer.[56,57] Despite this, a subset analysis of CALGB 9633 demonstrated improved survival using a carboplatin (Paraplatin)-based chemotherapy doublet, compared with observation alone, in patients with stage IB NSCLC greater than or equal to 4 cm.[5] This study was underpowered to detect a survival difference in all stage IB disease. As a result of this trial, carboplatin-based therapy is often used in patients with contraindications or expected intolerance to cisplatin. Head-to-head trials of cisplatin versus carboplatin in the adjuvant setting are lacking. A SEER-Medicare database suggested a similar benefit in both drugs in patients greater than the age of 65, with a suggestion of less toxicity with carboplatin.[58]

Neoadjuvant Chemotherapy

Neoadjuvant chemotherapy has shown similar 5-year overall survival when compared with adjuvant chemotherapy.[59] A clear overall survival benefit when compared with surgery alone, however, has been inconsistent in individual trials.[60–64] The NSCLC Meta-analysis Collaborative Group synthesized 15 randomized clinical trials and was able to identify an absolute survival improvement of 5% at 5 years,[65] similar to that found in the adjuvant trials. No particular regimen, number of drugs, or platinum agent appeared superior. As with the adjuvant meta-analyses, the benefit was similar regardless of age, gender, PS, histology, and clinical stage. As a result of these data, neoadjuvant chemotherapy is reasonable in patients with stage IB–IIIA NSCLC.

COMBINATION AND BIOLOGIC THERAPIES
Bevacizumab

The addition of bevacizumab (Avastin) to platinum-based chemotherapy has improved response rates and prolonged survival in patients with metastatic NSCLC.[66] Not surprisingly, efforts to use bevacizumab in the adjuvant and neoadjuvant settings have recently reached, or are nearing, completion. ECOG E1505 completed accrual of patients with resected stage IB–IIIA NSCLC receiving 1 of 4 cisplatin-based doublets, and randomized them to receive 1 year of adjuvant bevacizumab. Overall survival and progression-free survival were identical in both groups, however, consistent with a lack of benefit with the addition of bevacizumab.[67]

In the neoadjuvant setting, bevacizumab has shown a nonsignificant trend toward downstaging patients, but a definite benefit for therapy has not been realized.[68]

Epidermal Growth Factor Receptor Inhibitors and Other Biologic Agents

A retrospective series from Memorial Sloan Kettering Cancer Center explored the benefit of epidermal growth factor receptor (EGFR) tyrosine kinase inhibitors (TKIs) on patients with stage I–III resected lung adenocarcinoma with EGFR exon 19 deletions or exon 21 L858R mutations.[69] A statistically significant improvement in median disease-specific survival and a nonstatistically significant overall survival benefit was observed with the use of *EGFR* TKIs.

The RADIANT trial randomized patients with stage IB–IIIA NSCLC to erlotinib (Tarceva) or placebo for 2 years. Overall, patients randomized to erlotinib did not show a prolongation in disease-free survival. A suggestion of a benefit in the 16.5% of patients with an *EGFR* exon 19 deletion or exon 21 L858R mutations was erased with longer-term follow-up.[70,71]

The failure of erlotinib in the adjuvant setting leaves doubt as to the utility of other targeted agents and calls into question the importance of testing for EGFR, KRAS, ALK, ROS1, BRAF, RET, MET, and HER2 genetic alterations in early-stage NSCLC.

Immunotherapy

Immunotherapy in cancer treatment is currently a topic of widespread interest. The success of these therapies has been most significant in melanoma,[72] but immune checkpoint inhibitors have proven useful in metastatic NSCLC as well.[73,74]

Immunotherapy as adjuvant lung cancer treatment has been explored for decades, with little success.[75–77] A promising recent approach using the immunogenicity of the MAGE-A3 protein, expressed in 35% of tumors, unfortunately failed in a phase III trial.[78,79] The upcoming PEARLS trial (MK-3475-091/KEYNOTE-091) (NCT02504372) will examine the use of pembrolizumab (Keytruda) in the adjuvant setting.

TREATMENT OPTIONS AND COMPLICATIONS

Although the benefit of adjuvant chemotherapy has become clear, its toxicity is substantial and must be discussed with patients. The adverse effects of chemotherapeutic agents are diverse and often unique to a particular drug or drug class (**Table 3**). The use and perhaps dosing of a particular drug regimen should be tailored to the patient, with attention to the patient's medical history, physical impairments, and concomitant medications.

The platinum compounds cisplatin and carboplatin act like alkylating agents to halt cell division by forming cross-links to DNA, thereby preventing cell division and the completion of the cell cycle. Cisplatin should be avoided in patients with pre-existing kidney disease or hearing impairment, and caution should be used in those with peripheral neuropathy. Ototoxicity and nephrotoxicity are the most feared long-term toxicities, while nausea and vomiting may be severe. Carboplatin is primarily associated with myelosuppression, nausea, and vomiting. Drug interactions with phenytoin and warfarin must be considered.

The taxanes, paclitaxel, docetaxel, and nab-paclitaxel (Abraxane), are plant-based antineoplastic agents targeting the cellular microtubules, leading to cell death. The taxanes may cause peripheral neuropathy, hypersensitivity reactions, myelosuppression, alopecia, and fluid overload, to varying degrees.

Gemcitabine is classified as an antimetabolite that inhibits cellular division. Its common side effects include myelosuppression, fatigue, alopecia, and anorexia.

Mitomycin C is an antitumor antibiotic that acts during various phases of the cell cycle. It may cause myelosuppression, anorexia, fatigue, alopecia, nausea, and the rare but sometimes fatal thrombotic thrombocytopenic purpura/hemolytic-uremic syndrome.

The vinca alkaloids are derived from the periwinkle plant and function as antimicrotubule agents. Neuropathy, constipation, and myelosuppression are common toxic effects.

Table 3
Commonly used agents in adjuvant treatment of non–small cell lung cancer

Drug	Class	Mechanism of Action	Side Effects (>10% or Severe)
Cisplatin	Platinum	Alkylating agent	Nausea, kidney injury, hearing loss/tinnitus, electrolyte abnormalities, neuropathy, dysgeusia
Carboplatin	Platinum	Alkylating agent	Nausea, myelosuppression, peripheral neuropathy, abdominal pain, alopecia, dysgeusia
Paclitaxel	Taxane	Antineoplastic Agent	Neuropathy, myelosuppression, hypersensitivity infusion reactions, dyspnea, lethargy
Docetaxel	Taxane	Antineoplastic Agent	Myelosuppression, fluid retention, nausea, vomiting, muscle/joint/bone pain, nail change, alopecia
Gemcitabine	Antimetabolite	Nucleic acid synthesis inhibitor	Anorexia, myelosuppression, fatigue, nausea, dyspnea, insomnia
Mitomycin C	Antitumor antibiotic	Antineoplastic or Cytotoxic	Myelosuppression, hemolytic uremic syndrome, anorexia, nausea, hair loss, fatigue
Vinca alkaloids (vindesine, vinorelbine, vinblastine, vincristine)	Vinca alkaloid	Anti-microtubule agents: antineoplastic or cytotoxic	Alopecia, myelosuppression, constipation, abdominal cramps, weight loss, nausea, neuropathy, stomatitis, dysgeusia
Pemetrexed	Folate analogue	Disrupts folate-dependent metabolic processes essential for cell replication	Fatigue, myelosuppression, rash, liver function abnormalities, nausea, anorexia

Pemetrexed is an antifolate with a very low risk of alopecia, making it an attractive choice for patients with non-squamous cell lung cancer. Expected adverse effects include fatigue, nausea, anorexia, myelosuppression, and liver function abnormalities.

EVALUATION OF OUTCOME AND LONG-TERM RECOMMENDATIONS

Current guidelines by the National Comprehensive Cancer Network recommend history and physical examination accompanied by computed tomography (CT) of the chest with or without contrast every 6 to 12 months for 2 years, then noncontrast low-dose chest CT annually. CT imaging has been shown to be superior to chest radiograph, allowing for better detection of asymptomatic disease recurrence and the possibility of curative intervention.[80] A retrospective cohort study from the University of Pennsylvania suggests a correlation between the increase in CT surveillance and improvement in survival as this strategy became more widely adopted.[81]

PET/CT may have improved sensitivity in detection of recurrent disease,[82] but due to cost and resource concerns is generally reserved for patients with inconclusive findings on CT surveillance.

SUMMARY

When definitive local therapy is performed, early-stage NSCLC nevertheless carries a high risk of metastasis and mortality. The use of platinum-based adjuvant chemotherapy postoperatively improves long-term survival by approximately 5% or more across a wide range of histologic types and patient populations, including the elderly and those with comorbid disease. Although a survival benefit with chemotherapy for T1 disease has not been appreciated, patients with stage IB disease measuring at least 4 cm and those with locoregional lymph node involvement derive a benefit. Efforts to identify patients with or without an expected benefit based on individual disease biology and tumor genomics rather than stage are underway and appear promising.

ACKNOWLEDGMENTS

A special thanks to Shambavi Rao, Emory University, for her collaboration on this article.

REFERENCES

1. Howlader N, Noone AM, Krapcho M, et al. SEER cancer statistics review, 1975-2012, national cancer institute. Bethesda (MD): 2015. Available at: http://seer.cancer.gov/csr/1975_2012/. Accessed March 30, 2016.
2. Arriagada R, Bergman B, Dunant A, et al. Cisplatin-based adjuvant chemotherapy in patients with completely resected non-small-cell lung cancer. N Engl J Med 2004;350(4):351–60.
3. Winton T, Livingston R, Johnson D, et al. Vinorelbine plus cisplatin vs. observation in resected non-small-cell lung cancer. N Engl J Med 2005;352(25):2589–97.
4. Harpole DH Jr, Herndon JE 2nd, Young WG Jr, et al. Stage I nonsmall cell lung cancer. A multivariate analysis of treatment methods and patterns of recurrence. Cancer 1995;76(5):787–96.
5. Strauss GM, Herndon JE 2nd, Maddaus MA, et al. Adjuvant paclitaxel plus carboplatin compared with observation in stage IB non-small-cell lung cancer: CALGB 9633 with the Cancer and Leukemia Group B, Radiation Therapy

Oncology Group, and North Central Cancer Treatment Group study groups. J Clin Oncol 2008;26(31):5043–51.

6. Tsutani Y, Miyata Y, Kushitani K, et al. Propensity score-matched analysis of adjuvant chemotherapy for stage I non-small cell lung cancer. J Thorac Cardiovasc Surg 2014;148(4):1179–85.

7. Kiankhooy A, Taylor MD, LaPar DJ, et al. Predictors of early recurrence for node-negative t1 to t2b non-small cell lung cancer. Ann Thorac Surg 2014;98(4): 1175–83.

8. Fujimoto T, Cassivi SD, Yang P, et al. Completely resected N1 non-small cell lung cancer: factors affecting recurrence and long-term survival. J Thorac Cardiovasc Surg 2006;132(3):499–506.

9. Park SY, Lee JG, Kim J, et al. Efficacy of platinum-based adjuvant chemotherapy in T2aN0 stage IB non-small cell lung cancer. J Cardiothorac Surg 2013;8:151.

10. Consonni D, Pierobon M, Gail MH, et al. Lung cancer prognosis before and after recurrence in a population-based setting. J Natl Cancer Inst 2015;107(6): djv059.

11. Scagliotti GV, Parikh P, von Pawel J, et al. Phase III study comparing cisplatin plus gemcitabine with cisplatin plus pemetrexed in chemotherapy-naive patients with advanced-stage non-small-cell lung cancer. J Clin Oncol 2008;26(21):3543–51.

12. Scagliotti G, Brodowicz T, Shepherd FA, et al. Treatment-by-histology interaction analyses in three phase III trials show superiority of pemetrexed in nonsquamous non-small cell lung cancer. J Thorac Oncol 2011;6(1):64–70.

13. Yoshizawa A, Motoi N, Riely GJ, et al. Impact of proposed IASLC/ATS/ERS classification of lung adenocarcinoma: prognostic subgroups and implications for further revision of staging based on analysis of 514 stage I cases. Mod Pathol 2011;24(5):653–64.

14. Russell PA, Wainer Z, Wright GM, et al. Does lung adenocarcinoma subtype predict patient survival?: a clinicopathologic study based on the new International Association for the Study of Lung Cancer/American Thoracic Society/European Respiratory Society International Multidisciplinary Lung Adenocarcinoma classification. J Thorac Oncol 2011;6(9):1496–504.

15. Hung JJ, Yeh YC, Jeng WJ, et al. Predictive value of the International Association for the Study of Lung Cancer/American Thoracic Society/European Respiratory Society classification of lung adenocarcinoma in tumor recurrence and patient survival. J Clin Oncol 2014;32(22):2357–64.

16. Warth A, Muley T, Meister M, et al. The novel histologic International Association for the Study of Lung Cancer/American Thoracic Society/European Respiratory Society classification system of lung adenocarcinoma is a stage-independent predictor of survival. J Clin Oncol 2012;30(13):1438–46.

17. Ujiie H, Kadota K, Chaft JE, et al. Solid predominant histologic subtype in resected stage I lung adenocarcinoma is an independent predictor of early, extrathoracic, multisite recurrence and of poor postrecurrence survival. J Clin Oncol 2015;33(26):2877–84.

18. Tsao MS, Marguet S, Le Teuff G, et al. Subtype classification of lung adenocarcinoma predicts benefit from adjuvant chemotherapy in patients undergoing complete resection. J Clin Oncol 2015;33(30):3439–46.

19. Osarogiagbon RU, Lin CC, Smeltzer M, et al. Incomplete non-small-cell lung cancer (NSCLC) resections in the National Cancer Data Base (NCDB): predictors, prognosis and value of adjuvant therapy. ASCO Meeting Abstracts 2015; 33(15 Suppl):7527.

20. Olaussen KA, Dunant A, Fouret P, et al. DNA repair by ERCC1 in non-small-cell lung cancer and cisplatin-based adjuvant chemotherapy. N Engl J Med 2006; 355(10):983–91.

21. Wislez M, Barlesi F, Besse B, et al. Customized adjuvant phase II trial in patients with non-small-cell lung cancer: IFCT-0801 TASTE. J Clin Oncol 2014;32(12): 1256–61.

22. Lau A, Villeneuve NF, Sun Z, et al. Dual roles of Nrf2 in cancer. Pharmacol Res 2008;58(5–6):262–70.

23. Cescon DW, She D, Sakashita S, et al. NRF2 pathway activation and adjuvant chemotherapy benefit in lung squamous cell carcinoma. Clin Cancer Res 2015; 21(11):2499–505.

24. Tsao MS, Aviel-Ronen S, Ding K, et al. Prognostic and predictive importance of p53 and RAS for adjuvant chemotherapy in non small-cell lung cancer. J Clin Oncol 2007;25(33):5240–7.

25. Shepherd FA, Domerg C, Hainaut P, et al. Pooled analysis of the prognostic and predictive effects of KRAS mutation status and KRAS mutation subtype in early-stage resected non-small-cell lung cancer in four trials of adjuvant chemotherapy. J Clin Oncol 2013;31(17):2173–81.

26. Cuffe S, Bourredjem A, Graziano S, et al. A pooled exploratory analysis of the effect of tumor size and KRAS mutations on survival benefit from adjuvant platinum-based chemotherapy in node-negative non-small cell lung cancer. J Thorac Oncol 2012;7(6):963–72.

27. Dowsett M, Cuzick J, Wale C, et al. Prediction of risk of distant recurrence using the 21-gene recurrence score in node-negative and node-positive postmenopausal patients with breast cancer treated with anastrozole or tamoxifen: a Trans-ATAC study. J Clin Oncol 2010;28(11):1829–34.

28. Venook AP, Niedzwiecki D, Lopatin M, et al. Biologic determinants of tumor recurrence in stage II colon cancer: validation study of the 12-gene recurrence score in cancer and leukemia group B (CALGB) 9581. J Clin Oncol 2013;31(14): 1775–81.

29. Cooperberg MR, Simko JP, Cowan JE, et al. Validation of a cell-cycle progression gene panel to improve risk stratification in a contemporary prostatectomy cohort. J Clin Oncol 2013;31(11):1428–34.

30. Zhu CQ, Ding K, Strumpf D, et al. Prognostic and predictive gene signature for adjuvant chemotherapy in resected non-small-cell lung cancer. J Clin Oncol 2010;28(29):4417–24.

31. Der SD, Sykes J, Pintilie M, et al. Validation of a histology-independent prognostic gene signature for early-stage, non-small-cell lung cancer including stage IA patients. J Thorac Oncol 2014;9(1):59–64.

32. Wistuba II, Behrens C, Lombardi F, et al. Validation of a proliferation-based expression signature as prognostic marker in early stage lung adenocarcinoma. Clin Cancer Res 2013;19(22):6261–71.

33. Oxnard GR, Fidias P, Muzikansky A, et al. Non-small cell lung cancer in octogenarians: treatment practices and preferences. J Thorac Oncol 2007;2(11): 1029–35.

34. Thyss A, Saudes L, Otto J, et al. Renal tolerance of cisplatin in patients more than 80 years old. J Clin Oncol 1994;12(10):2121–5.

35. Fruh M, Rolland E, Pignon JP, et al. Pooled analysis of the effect of age on adjuvant cisplatin-based chemotherapy for completely resected non-small-cell lung cancer. J Clin Oncol 2008;26(21):3573–81.

36. Pepe C, Hasan B, Winton TL, et al. Adjuvant vinorelbine and cisplatin in elderly patients: National Cancer Institute of Canada and Intergroup Study JBR.10. J Clin Oncol 2007;25(12):1553–61.

37. Berry MF, Coleman BK, Curtis LH, et al. Benefit of adjuvant chemotherapy after resection of stage II (T1-2N1M0) non-small cell lung cancer in elderly patients. Ann Surg Oncol 2015;22(2):642–8.

38. Ganti AK, Williams CD, Gajra A, et al. Effect of age on the efficacy of adjuvant chemotherapy for resected non-small cell lung cancer. Cancer 2015;121(15): 2578–85.

39. Cuffe S, Booth CM, Peng Y, et al. Adjuvant chemotherapy for non-small-cell lung cancer in the elderly: a population-based study in Ontario, Canada. J Clin Oncol 2012;30(15):1813–21.

40. Burdett S, Pignon JP, Tierney J, et al. Adjuvant chemotherapy for resected early-stage non-small cell lung cancer. Cochrane Database Syst Rev 2015;(3):CD011430.

41. Tammemagi CM, Neslund-Dudas C, Simoff M, et al. Impact of comorbidity on lung cancer survival. Int J Cancer 2003;103(6):792–802.

42. Firat S, Bousamra M, Gore E, et al. Comorbidity and KPS are independent prognostic factors in stage I non-small-cell lung cancer. Int J Radiat Oncol Biol Phys 2002;52(4):1047–57.

43. Pignon JP, Tribodet H, Scagliotti GV, et al. Lung adjuvant cisplatin evaluation: a pooled analysis by the LACE collaborative group. J Clin Oncol 2008;26(21): 3552–9.

44. Parsons A, Daley A, Begh R, et al. Influence of smoking cessation after diagnosis of early stage lung cancer on prognosis: systematic review of observational studies with meta-analysis. BMJ 2010;340:b5569.

45. Zhang J, Kamdar O, Le W, et al. Nicotine induces resistance to chemotherapy by modulating mitochondrial signaling in lung cancer. Am J Respir Cell Mol Biol 2009;40(2):135–46.

46. Tammemagi CM, Neslund-Dudas C, Simoff M, et al. In lung cancer patients, age, race-ethnicity, gender and smoking predict adverse comorbidity, which in turn predicts treatment and survival. J Clin Epidemiol 2004;57(6):597–609.

47. Sardari Nia P, Weyler J, Colpaert C, et al. Prognostic value of smoking status in operated non-small cell lung cancer. Lung Cancer 2005;47(3):351–9.

48. Booth CM, Shepherd FA, Peng Y, et al. Time to adjuvant chemotherapy and survival in non-small cell lung cancer: a population-based study. Cancer 2013; 119(6):1243–50.

49. Ramsden K, Laskin J, Ho C. Adjuvant chemotherapy in resected stage II non-small cell lung cancer: evaluating the impact of dose intensity and time to treatment. Clin Oncol (R Coll Radiol) 2015;27(7):394–400.

50. Butts CA, Ding K, Seymour L, et al. Randomized phase III trial of vinorelbine plus cisplatin compared with observation in completely resected stage IB and II non-small-cell lung cancer: updated survival analysis of JBR-10. J Clin Oncol 2010; 28(1):29–34.

51. Douillard JY, Rosell R, De Lena M, et al. Adjuvant vinorelbine plus cisplatin versus observation in patients with completely resected stage IB-IIIA non-small-cell lung cancer (Adjuvant Navelbine International Trialist Association [ANITA]): a randomised controlled trial. Lancet Oncol 2006;7(9):719–27.

52. Scagliotti GV, Fossati R, Torri V, et al. Randomized study of adjuvant chemotherapy for completely resected stage I, II, or IIIA non-small-cell lung cancer. J Natl Cancer Inst 2003;95(19):1453–61.

53. Waller D, Peake MD, Stephens RJ, et al. Chemotherapy for patients with non-small cell lung cancer: the surgical setting of the Big Lung Trial. Eur J Cardio-thorac Surg 2004;26(1):173–82.

54. Kreuter M, Vansteenkiste J, Fischer JR, et al. Randomized phase 2 trial on refinement of early-stage NSCLC adjuvant chemotherapy with cisplatin and pemetrexed versus cisplatin and vinorelbine: the TREAT study. Ann Oncol 2013;24(4):986–92.

55. Miksad RA, Gonen M, Lynch TJ, et al. Interpreting trial results in light of conflicting evidence: a Bayesian analysis of adjuvant chemotherapy for non-small-cell lung cancer. J Clin Oncol 2009;27(13):2245–52.

56. Ardizzoni A, Boni L, Tiseo M, et al. Cisplatin- versus carboplatin-based chemotherapy in first-line treatment of advanced non-small-cell lung cancer: an individual patient data meta-analysis. J Natl Cancer Inst 2007;99(11):847–57.

57. Hotta K, Matsuo K, Ueoka H, et al. Meta-analysis of randomized clinical trials comparing cisplatin to carboplatin in patients with advanced non-small-cell lung cancer. J Clin Oncol 2004;22(19):3852–9.

58. Gu F, Strauss GM, Wisnivesky JP. Platinum-based adjuvant chemotherapy (ACT) in elderly patients with non-small cell lung cancer (NSCLC) in the SEER-Medicare database: comparison between carboplatin- and cisplatin-based regimens. ASCO Meeting Abstracts 2011;29(15 Suppl):7014.

59. Felip E, Rosell R, Maestre JA, et al. Preoperative chemotherapy plus surgery versus surgery plus adjuvant chemotherapy versus surgery alone in early-stage non-small-cell lung cancer. J Clin Oncol 2010;28(19):3138–45.

60. Gilligan D, Nicolson M, Smith I, et al. Preoperative chemotherapy in patients with resectable non-small cell lung cancer: results of the MRC LU22/NVALT 2/EORTC 08012 multicentre randomised trial and update of systematic review. Lancet 2007;369(9577):1929–37.

61. Rosell R, Gomez-Codina J, Camps C, et al. A randomized trial comparing preoperative chemotherapy plus surgery with surgery alone in patients with non-small-cell lung cancer. N Engl J Med 1994;330(3):153–8.

62. Depierre A, Milleron B, Moro-Sibilot D, et al. Preoperative chemotherapy followed by surgery compared with primary surgery in resectable stage I (except T1N0), II, and IIIa non-small-cell lung cancer. J Clin Oncol 2002;20(1):247–53.

63. Roth JA, Fossella F, Komaki R, et al. A randomized trial comparing perioperative chemotherapy and surgery with surgery alone in resectable stage IIIA non-small-cell lung cancer. J Natl Cancer Inst 1994;86(9):673–80.

64. Pisters KM, Vallieres E, Crowley JJ, et al. Surgery with or without preoperative paclitaxel and carboplatin in early-stage non-small-cell lung cancer: Southwest Oncology Group Trial S9900, an intergroup, randomized, phase III trial. J Clin Oncol 2010;28(11):1843–9.

65. NSCLC Meta-analysis Collaborative Group. Preoperative chemotherapy for non-small-cell lung cancer: a systematic review and meta-analysis of individual participant data. Lancet 2014;383(9928):1561–71.

66. Sandler A, Gray R, Perry MC, et al. Paclitaxel-carboplatin alone or with bevacizumab for non-small-cell lung cancer. N Engl J Med 2006;355(24):2542–50.

67. Wakelee HA, Dahlberg SE, Keller SM, et al. Randomized phase III trial of adjuvant chemotherapy with or without bevacizumab in resected non-small cell lung cancer (NSCLC): results of E1505 (abstract 1608) randomized phase III trial of adjuvant chemotherapy with or without bevacizumab in resected non-small cell lung cancer (NSCLC): results of E1505. 16th World Conference on Lung Cancer. Denver, Colorado, September 2015.

68. Chaft JE, Rusch V, Ginsberg MS, et al. Phase II trial of neoadjuvant bevacizumab plus chemotherapy and adjuvant bevacizumab in patients with resectable non-squamous non-small-cell lung cancers. J Thorac Oncol 2013;8(8):1084–90.
69. D'Angelo SP, Janjigian YY, Ahye N, et al. Distinct clinical course of EGFR-mutant resected lung cancers: results of testing of 1118 surgical specimens and effects of adjuvant gefitinib and erlotinib. J Thorac Oncol 2012;7(12):1815–22.
70. O'Brien MER, Kelly K, Altorki NK, et al. Final follow-up (F/U) results from RADIANT: a randomized double blind phase 3 trial of adjuvant erlotinib (E) versus placebo (P) following complete tumor resection in patients (pts) with stage IB-IIIA EGFR positive (IHC/FISH) non-small cell lung cancer (NSCLC). ASCO Meeting Abstracts 2015;33(15 Suppl):7540.
71. Kelly K, Altorki NK, Eberhardt WE, et al. Adjuvant erlotinib versus placebo in patients with stage IB-IIIA non-small-cell lung cancer (RADIANT): a randomized, double-blind, phase III trial. J Clin Oncol 2015;33(34):4007–14.
72. Larkin J, Chiarion-Sileni V, Gonzalez R, et al. Combined nivolumab and ipilimumab or monotherapy in untreated melanoma. N Engl J Med 2015;373(1): 23–34.
73. Brahmer J, Reckamp KL, Baas P, et al. Nivolumab versus docetaxel in advanced squamous-cell non-small-cell lung cancer. N Engl J Med 2015;373(2):123–35.
74. Garon EB, Rizvi NA, Hui R, et al. Pembrolizumab for the treatment of non-small-cell lung cancer. N Engl J Med 2015;372(21):2018–28.
75. Yamamura Y, Sakatani M, Ogura T, et al. Adjuvant immunotherapy of lung cancer with BCG cell wall skeleton (BCG-CWS). Cancer 1979;43(4):1314–9.
76. Lee YC, Luh SP, Wu RM, et al. Adjuvant immunotherapy with intrapleural streptococcus pyogenes (OK-432) in lung cancer patients after resection. Cancer Immunol Immunother 1994;39(4):269–74.
77. Fox RM, Woods RL, Tattersall MH, et al. A randomized study of adjuvant immunotherapy with levamisole and corynebacterium parvum in operable non-small cell lung cancer. Int J Radiat Oncol Biol Phys 1980;6(8):1043–5.
78. Pujol JL, Vansteenkiste JF, De Pas TM, et al. Safety and immunogenicity of MAGE-A3 cancer immunotherapeutic with or without adjuvant chemotherapy in patients with resected stage IB to III MAGE-A3-positive NSCLC. J Thorac Oncol 2015;10(10):1458–67.
79. Vansteenkiste J, Zielinski M, Linder A, et al. Adjuvant MAGE-A3 immunotherapy in resected non-small-cell lung cancer: phase II randomized study results. J Clin Oncol 2013;31(19):2396–403.
80. Hanna WC, Paul NS, Darling GE, et al. Minimal-dose computed tomography is superior to chest x-ray for the follow-up and treatment of patients with resected lung cancer. J Thorac Cardiovasc Surg 2014;147(1):30–3.
81. Ciunci CA, Paulson EC, Mitra N, et al. Patterns and effectiveness of surveillance after curative intent surgery in stage I-IIIA non-small cell lung cancer. ASCO Meeting Abstracts 2015;33(15 Suppl):7546.
82. Dane B, Grechushkin V, Plank A, et al. PET/CT vs. non-contrast CT alone for surveillance 1-year post lobectomy for stage I non-small-cell lung cancer. Am J Nucl Med Mol Imaging 2013;3(5):408–16.
83. Strauss GM, Wang XF, Maddaus M, et al. Adjuvant chemotherapy (AC) in stage IB non-small cell lung cancer (NSCLC): long-term follow-up of cancer and leukemia group B (CALGB) 9633. ASCO Meeting Abstracts 2011;29(15 Suppl):7015.

Targeted Therapy and Immunotherapy for Lung Cancer

 CrossMark

Evan C. Naylor, MD*, Jatin K. Desani, MD, Paul K. Chung, MD

KEYWORDS

• Molecular • Targeted therapy • Immunotherapy • Non–small cell lung cancer

KEY POINTS

- Targeted therapy and immunotherapy have had an increasing role in the management of patients with advanced non–small cell lung cancer (NSCLC).
- Therapies targeting patients with epidermal growth factor receptor (EGFR) mutations and anaplastic lymphoma kinase (ALK) rearrangements have proved most successful, whereas others specific for additional genetic alterations seem promising.
- Immunotherapy in lung cancer, primarily through checkpoint inhibition, permits the activation of tumor-specific T cells often suppressed by cancer cells.
- Adverse effects of these drugs are often mild and manageable, improving quality of life and limiting cumulative toxicity seen with use of cytotoxic chemotherapy.

INTRODUCTION

The management of patients with advanced NSCLC has evolved dramatically over the past decade. Therapeutic options were previously limited to cytotoxic chemotherapy in a 1-size-fits-all approach. As more information becomes known about the driving molecular events behind tumorigenesis, however, researchers are designing drugs capable of interfering with these events in a more individualized approach. The first such drugs in NSCLC were the targeted agents, biologic compounds that interact with cell surface receptors or their downstream partners critical in cancer development. These agents have shown a monumental benefit in a small number of patients with NSCLC. The more recent addition has been the immunotherapeutic agents, which seem to have a broader benefit and are providing durable responses in NSCLC not previously seen.

The authors have nothing to disclose.
Hematology and Oncology, Southern Ocean Medical Center, Meridian Cancer Care, 1140 Route 72 West, Manahawkin, NJ 08050, USA
* Corresponding author.
E-mail address: enaylor@meridianhealth.com

Surg Oncol Clin N Am 25 (2016) 601–609
http://dx.doi.org/10.1016/j.soc.2016.02.011
surgonc.theclinics.com

TARGETED AGENTS
Background

Several genetic alterations have been identified as drivers of tumorigenesis in NSCLC. Among the most important described in lung cancer is the ERK-MAPK cascade. In this cascade, activating mutations in EGFR, RAS, and BRAF found in lung cancer lead to malignant transformation and gene expression changes.[1] Patients with KRAS-mutant tumors, accounting for 25% of cases of adenocarcinoma, are often predictive of a lack of benefit of tyrosine kinase inhibitors (TKIs)[2] and associated with poorer overall survival.[3]

The number of therapeutic targets is rapidly growing. Fortunately, the drugs being developed for these targets generally have more favorable toxicity profiles than cytotoxic chemotherapy (**Table 1**).

Epidermal Growth Factor Receptor Mutations

The cell surface receptor EGFR, when dimerized, activates tyrosine kinases. This action contributes to control of normal cell proliferation, angiogenesis, adhesion, motility, and apoptosis. Loss of this control contributes to the malignant potential of a lung cancer cell.

Mutations in EGFR account for 15% of lung adenocarcinoma in the United States, the most common of which occur in exon 19 (exon 19del) and exon 21 (L858R). Women and nonsmokers have a slightly higher likelihood of mutations. The frequency

Table 1
Select targeted biologic agents in non–small cell lung cancer

Class	Drugs	Adverse Effects
EGFR inhibitors	Erlotinib, afatinib, gefitinib, osimertinib, rociletinib	Rash, diarrhea, anorexia, fatigue, dyspnea, cough, nausea, vomiting, interstitial lung disease, hepatotoxicity
ALK inhibitors	Crizotinib, ceritinib, brigatinib, alectinib	Vision disorder, diarrhea, edema, transaminase elevations, vomiting, constipation, dysgeusia, fatigue, pyrexia, pain in extremity, headache, dizziness, pneumonitis
BRAF inhibitors	Vemurafenib, dabrafenib	Other malignancies, hypersensitivity reactions, dermatologic reactions, QT prolongation, hepatotoxicity, uveitis, radiation recall/sensitivity, arthralgia, rash, alopecia, photosensitivity, nausea, pruritis
MEK inhibitors	Trametinib, cobimetinib	Hemorrhage, rash, cardiomyopathy, hepatotoxicity, retinopathy and retinal vein occlusion, rhabdomyolysis, diarrhea, photosensitivity, nausea, pyrexia, vomiting
HER2-blocking antibodies	Trastuzumab	Headache, diarrhea, nausea, chills, cardiomyopathy, infusion reactions, pulmonary toxicity
Multitargeted kinase inhibitors	Cabozantinib	Gastrointestinal perforation/fistula, hemorrhage, thrombotic events, wound complications, hypertension, hand-foot syndrome, osteonecrosis of the jaw, proteinuria, diarrhea, stomatitis, weight loss, anorexia, dysgeusia, nausea, fatigue

of EGFR mutations in various Asian populations increases to 22% to 62% of NSCLCs.[4]

Four EGFR TKIs, erlotinib (Tarceva), gefitinib (Iressa), afatinib (Gilotrif), and osimertinib (Tagrisso), are currently Food and Drug Administration (FDA) approved and in clinical use in the United States. Compared with standard cytotoxic chemotherapy doublets, this class of drugs has proved to prolong progression-free survival (PFS) in patients with advanced NSCLC with activating EGFR mutations.

Gefitinib showed an impressive improvement in PFS compared with carboplatin (Paraplatin) and paclitaxel (Taxol) in the Iressa Pan-Asia Study trial in 2009. In this study, PFS was doubled with gefitinib at 10.8 months compared with 5.4 months for the standard cytotoxic chemotherapy doublet.[5] This study enrolled unselected Asian patients with a higher frequency of EGFR mutations than that seen in a Western population. Despite these impressive results and its extensive clinical use in Asia, gefitinib use has been limited in the United States until FDA approval in 2015. Gefitinib is approved for patients whose tumor contains an EGFR exon 19 deletion or exon 21 L858R.

Erlotinib was also compared with standard cytotoxic chemotherapy in clinical trials. In the OPTIMAL trial, an impressive improvement in PFS of 8 months was noted when erlotinib was compared with gemcitabine (Gemzar) plus carboplatin.[6] Similar improvements in PFS of 5 to 6 months were found in the EURTAC[7] and ENSURE[8] trials. Despite these improvements in PFS, no statistically significant difference in overall survival was found in either trial comparing erlotinib to standard cytotoxic chemotherapy, likely due to crossover of therapy after progression.

Afatinib is as an oral irreversible inhibitor of EGFR and HER2. In the LUX-Lung 3 trial, afatinib showed a significant increase in PFS of 6.7 months compared with cisplatin (Platinol) and pemetrexed (Alimta) in treatment-naïve patients with EGFR exon 19 deletions and L858R point mutations.[9] Notably, 4 treatment-related deaths were seen with afatinib as opposed to none with chemotherapy. Afatinib is FDA approved for first-line treatment of patients with metastatic NSCLC whose tumors have EGFR exon 19 deletions or exon 21 substitution mutations. Activity after failure of erlotinib or gefitinib is limited, with only a 7% response rate.[10]

An EGFR T790M mutation in exon 20 is associated with acquired resistance to TKI therapy and has been reported in up to 63% of patients with disease progression after initial response to front-line TKIs.[11,12] Osimertinib and rociletinib are third-generation EGFR inhibitors active in preclinical models of EGFR T790M-mutated NSCLC. In separate studies of patients whose disease had progressed on EGFR-directed therapy, the objective response rate among T790M-positive disease was approximately 60% and the rate among patients with T790M-negative disease was 20% to 30%.[13,14]

EML4-ALK Translocations

Translocation of ALK and Echinoderm Microtubule-Associated Protein-Like 4 (EML4) from an inversion of the short arm of chromosome 2 results in a fusion protein EML4-ALK that activates several pathways driving cell survival and proliferation.[15] These translocations are present in 3% to 5% of NSCLC patients and define a distinct subset of lung cancer patients.[16]

Crizotinib (Xalkori) is an oral inhibitor of ALK, MET, and ROS1 kinases. In patients with treatment-naïve advanced ALK-positive NSCLC in PROFILE 1014, crizotinib performed better than cytotoxic chemotherapy, with median PFS of 10.9 months versus 7.0 months, a response rate of 74% versus 45%, and improvements in lung cancer symptoms and quality of life.[17] Overall survival was not significantly different, likely owing to a 70% crossover rate on progression in the chemotherapy arm.

Ceritinib (Zykadia) produces a high response rate of 55.4% in patients previously treated with crizotinib and 69.5% in patients naïve to ALK inhibitors.[18] Patients with prior exposure had a meaningful 6.9 month PFS on ceritinib. Two other ALK inhibitors, brigatinib (AP26113) and alectinib (Alecensa), have also shown promising activity in patients with progression on crizotinib, including patients with brain metastases.[19,20]

ROS1 Rearrangements

ROS1 is a tyrosine kinase receptor of the insulin receptor family. At least 12 different partner proteins form fusions with ROS1, producing constitutive kinase activity, thereby driving cellular transformation.[21,22] Rearrangements of ROS1 are found in 1% to 2% of NSCLC specimens and are more common in patients with a light or no smoking history and those with adenocarcinoma.

Crizotinib has been shown to induce responses in vitro and in limited experience in patients with ROS1 rearrangements.[21] A recent phase I clinical trial supported these data, showing a high response rate of 72%, with 6% of patients achieving complete responses.[23] Furthermore, median PFS was 19.2 months, and all ROS1 fusions showed a benefit.

BRAF V600 Mutations

BRAF mutations are identified in approximately 2% of lung adenocarcinoma tumors.[24] Twenty patients with NSCLC harboring a V600 mutation received treatment with vemurafenib (Zelboraf), resulting in a 42% response rate in evaluable patients and a median PFS of 7.3 months.[25] Dabrafenib (Tafinlar) also demonstrated activity in 17 patients with BRAF V600E mutations, with an overall response rate of 54%.[26] A retrospective study of patients with BRAF mutations revealed a similar response rate of 53% and PFS of 5 months in patients treated with various BRAF inhibitors.[24]

Combination therapy with dabrafenib and trametinib (Mekinist) yielded an impressive 63% response rate in 24 evaluable NSCLC patients harboring a BRAF V600E mutation.[27]

MET Amplification or Exon 14 Skipping Mutation

The proto-oncogene MET, also known as hepatocyte growth factor receptor, is involved in signal transduction. MET exon 14 splice site alterations and other mutations have been shown to result in exon skipping and MET activation and are present in approximately 3% of lung adenocarcinoma and 2.3% of other lung neoplasms.[28] These alterations result in tumor cell proliferation, invasion, and metastasis.

A phase I study of patients with MET-amplified NSCLC treated with crizotinib revealed a response rate of 33%, perhaps better in those with high amplification, defined as MET/CEP7 ratio of 5 or greater.[29] Those harboring MET exon 14 skipping mutations have shown responses to both crizotinib and cabozantinib.[30] Additionally, the investigational MET inhibitor capmatinib (INC280) induced partial responses in several patients in phase I clinical trials.[28]

RET Rearrangements

Rearrangements or fusions of RET, a proto-oncogene encoding a tyrosine kinase involved in extracellular signaling, are identified in 1% to 2% of NSCLCs, primarily adenocarcinoma in nonsmokers.[31] Twenty patients with adenocarcinoma harboring RET rearrangements were treated in a phase II open-label trial with the multi-TKI cabozantinib (Cometriq). The investigators noted an overall response rate of 28% and stable disease in 72%.[31] Median PFS was 7 months.

HER2 Mutations

HER2 mutations are the driver mutations found in approximately 2% of NSCLCs. These mutations are primarily found in women, never-smokers, and almost exclusively adenocarcinoma histology. In-frame insertions in exon 20 lead to constitutive activation of the HER2 receptor, and its downstream signaling pathways, in turn driving neoplastic transformation.

Trastuzumab (Herceptin) and afatinib have yielded partial responses and disease control in patients with HER2-mutated NSCLC.[32,33]

Recommended Testing

Based on these data, the National Comprehensive Cancer Network guidelines for NSCLC (version 2.2016) recommend all patients with metastatic NSCLC of histologic subtypes adenocarcinoma, large cell carcinoma, and NSCLC not otherwise specified be tested for EGFR mutations and ALK rearrangement as part of broad molecular profiling. Patients with squamous cell carcinoma can be considered for testing, especially in never-smokers, mixed histology, or small biopsy specimens. At this time, the data do not support routine testing of patients treated with curative intent. The College of American Pathologists recommends routine testing for all patients, including resectable NSCLC.

IMMUNOTHERAPY
Background

The programmed cell death-1 receptor (PD-1) is found on cytotoxic T cells and T-regulatory cells and is expressed when T cells become activated in response to inflammation or infection in peripheral tissues. Binding of the PD-1 ligand to its receptor inactivates the T cell to limit the immune response to the stimuli, thus causing an immune suppression.[34]

Cancer cells express PD-1, allowing them to be hidden from natural immune attack. Anti–PD-1 therapies disrupt this pathway by preventing the PD-1 ligand from binding to its receptor, leaving activated cytotoxic T cells available to attack the cancer cells. Immunotherapies directed at PD-1 or its ligand, PD-L1, have demonstrated efficacy in both nonsquamous and squamous cell NSCLCs.

PD-1/PD-L1 Inhibitors

CheckMate 063 was a phase II single-arm trial of nivolumab (Opdivo) in 117 patients with stage IIIB or stage IV squamous cell NSCLC that had progressed on at least 2 prior treatment regimens.[35] Median PFS was 1.9 months and median overall survival was 8.2 months. Although responses were seen in both patient subgroups, those with at least 5% PD-L1 positivity had numerically higher rates of partial response (24% vs 14%) and lower rates of progressive disease (44% vs 49%) compared with those with less than 5% PD-L1 positivity.

CheckMate 017 was a phase III randomized trial comparing standard docetaxel with nivolumab in 272 patients with stage IIIB or stage IV squamous cell NSCLC who failed only 1 prior platinum-containing treatment.[36] Median overall survival was 9.2 months with nivolumab, compared with 6.0 months with docetaxel, with a 41% reduction in the risk of death on the nivolumab arm. Objective response was also significantly higher on the nivolumab arm compared with docetaxel. In this trial, no level of PD-L1 positivity by IHC staining (1%, 5%, and 10% levels were evaluated) predicted response or was prognostic for survival.

Pembrolizumab (Keytruda), an anti–PD-L1 monoclonal antibody, was evaluated in the phase I KEYNOTE-001 trial in 495 patients who were either treatment naïve or treatment experienced with any histologic type of stage IIIB or stage IV NSCLC to determine the preliminary safety and efficacy of pembrolizumab in this population.[37] The overall response rate was 19.4%. Previously untreated patients were more likely to respond to therapy (25% vs 18%) and had longer median duration of response (23.3 months vs 10.4 months) than those previously treated. No difference was seen in the response rate based on histologic subtype (squamous vs nonsquamous). Current and former smokers had higher response rates (22.5%) compared with never-smokers (10.3%). Median overall survival was longer for patients receiving pembrolizumab as first-line therapy (16.2 months) compared with those receiving pembrolizumab after failing at least 1 prior regimen (9.3 months). Tumors with more than 50% PD-L1 expression had an overall response rate of 45.2%.

The minimum level of PD-L1 expression necessary to predict treatment response with anti–PD-1 therapies is unknown. Tumors with PD-L1 expression, however, have higher response rates across various tumor types, although those testing negative for PD-L1 also respond to these therapies.[38]

In addition to nivolumab and permbrolizumab, several other immune checkpoint inhibitors are in late-stage development. PD-L1 inhibitors under investigation are atezolizumab (MPDL3280A),[39] durvalumab (MEDI4736), avelumab (MSB0010718C), and BMS-936559. These drugs generally have a favorable adverse effect profile (**Table 2**).

CTLA-4 Inhibitors

In a randomized phase II trial with untreated advanced NSCLC, ipilimumab (Yervoy) or placebo in combination with carboplatin and paclitaxel, either concurrent or phased (starting after 2 cycles of chemotherapy), showed improvement in phased ipilimumab over placebo but not concurrent ipilimumab.[40] Phased ipilimumab had an improved overall response rate (32% vs 21% and 18%) and median overall survival (12.2 months vs 9.7 months and 8.3 months) compared with concurrent ipilimumab and placebo. In the phased ipilimumab arm, the overall survival advantage was limited to squamous histology. As a result of this study, this chemoimmunotherapy combination is now in phase III testing for patients with squamous NSCLC (NCT01285609). Ipilimumab has also shown modest response rates in conjunction with nivolumab.[41]

Future Directions

There are several ongoing studies of immune checkpoint inhibitors as single agents or in combination with chemotherapeutic agents seeking to expand their therapeutic indications to adjuvant or maintenance therapy. The use of immunotherapy in early-stage or locally advanced disease is currently not supported by the literature.

Table 2		
Select immunotherapeutic agents in lung cancer		
Class	**Drugs**	**Adverse Effects**
PD-1– or PD-L1–blocking antibodies	Nivolumab, pembrolizumab, atezolizumab (MPDL3280A), durvalumab (MEDI4736), avelumab (MSB0010718C), BMS-936559	Fatigue, nausea, anorexia, colitis, hepatitis, pneumonitis, endocrinopathies, nephritis, rash, encephalitis
CTLA4-blocking antibodies	Ipilimumab	Fatigue, rash, diarrhea, colitis, endocrinopathies, hepatitis

SUMMARY/DISCUSSION

New therapies have recently transformed the management of advanced lung cancer. By targeting molecules driving malignant growth, these treatments largely spare normal cells. In select patients, targeted agents and immunotherapies provide a meaningful improvement in survival over conventional cytotoxic chemotherapeutic agents. In addition, these drugs are often more tolerable, improving quality of life and permitting long-term use. The benefit, however, has not yet translated to earlier stages of disease or in conjunction with other modalities.

REFERENCES

1. Roberts PJ, Der CJ. Targeting the raf-MEK-ERK mitogen-activated protein kinase cascade for the treatment of cancer. Oncogene 2007;26(22):3291–310.
2. Eberhard DA, Johnson BE, Amler LC, et al. Mutations in the epidermal growth factor receptor and in KRAS are predictive and prognostic indicators in patients with non-small-cell lung cancer treated with chemotherapy alone and in combination with erlotinib. J Clin Oncol 2005;23(25):5900–9.
3. Roberts PJ, Stinchcombe TE. KRAS mutation: should we test for it, and does it matter? J Clin Oncol 2013;31(8):1112–21.
4. Shi Y, Au JS, Thongprasert S, et al. A prospective, molecular epidemiology study of EGFR mutations in asian patients with advanced non-small-cell lung cancer of adenocarcinoma histology (PIONEER). J Thorac Oncol 2014;9(2):154–62.
5. Maemondo M, Inoue A, Kobayashi K, et al. Gefitinib or chemotherapy for non-small-cell lung cancer with mutated EGFR. N Engl J Med 2010;362(25):2380–8.
6. Zhou C, Wu YL, Chen G, et al. Final overall survival results from a randomised, phase III study of erlotinib versus chemotherapy as first-line treatment of EGFR mutation-positive advanced non-small-cell lung cancer (OPTIMAL, CTONG-0802). Ann Oncol 2015;26(9):1877–83.
7. Rosell R, Carcereny E, Gervais R, et al. Erlotinib versus standard chemotherapy as first-line treatment for european patients with advanced EGFR mutation-positive non-small-cell lung cancer (EURTAC): a multicentre, open-label, randomised phase 3 trial. Lancet Oncol 2012;13(3):239–46.
8. Wu YL, Zhou C, Liam CK, et al. First-line erlotinib versus gemcitabine/cisplatin in patients with advanced EGFR mutation-positive non-small-cell lung cancer: analyses from the phase III, randomized, open-label, ENSURE study. Ann Oncol 2015;26(9):1883–9.
9. Sequist LV, Yang JC, Yamamoto N, et al. Phase III study of afatinib or cisplatin plus pemetrexed in patients with metastatic lung adenocarcinoma with EGFR mutations. J Clin Oncol 2013;31(27):3327–34.
10. Miller VA, Hirsh V, Cadranel J, et al. Afatinib versus placebo for patients with advanced, metastatic non-small-cell lung cancer after failure of erlotinib, gefitinib, or both, and one or two lines of chemotherapy (LUX-lung 1): a phase 2b/3 randomised trial. Lancet Oncol 2012;13(5):528–38.
11. Onitsuka T, Uramoto H, Nose N, et al. Acquired resistance to gefitinib: the contribution of mechanisms other than the T790M, MET, and HGF status. Lung Cancer 2010;68(2):198–203.
12. Yu HA, Arcila ME, Rekhtman N, et al. Analysis of tumor specimens at the time of acquired resistance to EGFR-TKI therapy in 155 patients with EGFR-mutant lung cancers. Clin Cancer Res 2013;19(8):2240–7.
13. Sequist LV, Soria JC, Goldman JW, et al. Rociletinib in EGFR-mutated non-small-cell lung cancer. N Engl J Med 2015;372(18):1700–9.

14. Janne PA, Yang JC, Kim DW, et al. AZD9291 in EGFR inhibitor-resistant non-small-cell lung cancer. N Engl J Med 2015;372(18):1689–99.

15. Shaw AT, Solomon B. Targeting anaplastic lymphoma kinase in lung cancer. Clin Cancer Res 2011;17(8):2081–6.

16. Soda M, Choi YL, Enomoto M, et al. Identification of the transforming EML4-ALK fusion gene in non-small-cell lung cancer. Nature 2007;448(7153):561–6.

17. Solomon BJ, Mok T, Kim DW, et al. First-line crizotinib versus chemotherapy in ALK-positive lung cancer. N Engl J Med 2014;371(23):2167–77.

18. Kim D, Mehra R, Tan DS, et al. Ceritinib in advanced anaplastic lymphoma kinase (ALK)-rearranged (ALK+) non-small cell lung cancer (NSCLC): results of the ASCEND-1 trial. ASCO Meet Abstr 2014;32(Suppl 15):8003.

19. Camidge DR, Bazhenova L, Salgia R, et al. Safety and efficacy of brigatinib (AP26113) in advanced malignancies, including ALK+ non-small cell lung cancer (NSCLC). ASCO Meet Abstr 2015;33(Suppl 15):8062.

20. Gandhi L, Shaw A, Gadgeel SM, et al. A phase II, open-label, multicenter study of the ALK inhibitor alectinib in an ALK+ non-small-cell lung cancer (NSCLC) U.S./canadian population who had progressed on crizotinib (NP28761). ASCO Meet Abstr 2015;33(Suppl 15):8019.

21. Bergethon K, Shaw AT, Ou SH, et al. ROS1 rearrangements define a unique molecular class of lung cancers. J Clin Oncol 2012;30(8):863–70.

22. Davies KD, Doebele RC. Molecular pathways: ROS1 fusion proteins in cancer. Clin Cancer Res 2013;19(15):4040–5.

23. Shaw AT, Ou SH, Bang YJ, et al. Crizotinib in ROS1-rearranged non-small-cell lung cancer. N Engl J Med 2014;371(21):1963–71.

24. Gautschi O, Milia J, Cabarrou B, et al. Targeted therapy for patients with BRAF-mutant lung cancer: results from the european EURAF cohort. J Thorac Oncol 2015;10(10):1451–7.

25. Hyman DM, Puzanov I, Subbiah V, et al. Vemurafenib in multiple nonmelanoma cancers with BRAF V600 mutations. N Engl J Med 2015;373(8):726–36.

26. Planchard D, Mazieres J, Riely GJ, et al. Interim results of phase II study BRF113928 of dabrafenib in BRAF V600E mutation-positive non-small cell lung cancer (NSCLC) patients. ASCO Meet Abstr 2013;31(Suppl 15):8009.

27. Planchard D, Groen HJM, Kim TM, et al. Interim results of a phase II study of the BRAF inhibitor (BRAFi) dabrafenib (D) in combination with the MEK inhibitor trametinib (T) in patients (pts) with BRAF V600E mutated (mut) metastatic non-small cell lung cancer (NSCLC). ASCO Meet Abstr 2015;33(Suppl 15):8006.

28. Frampton GM, Ali SM, Rosenzweig M, et al. Activation of MET via diverse exon 14 splicing alterations occurs in multiple tumor types and confers clinical sensitivity to MET inhibitors. Cancer Discov 2015;5(8):850–9.

29. Camidge DR, Ou SI, Shapiro G, et al. Efficacy and safety of crizotinib in patients with advanced c-MET-amplified non-small cell lung cancer (NSCLC). ASCO Meet Abstr 2014;32(Suppl 15):8001.

30. Paik PK, Drilon A, Fan PD, et al. Response to MET inhibitors in patients with stage IV lung adenocarcinomas harboring MET mutations causing exon 14 skipping. Cancer Discov 2015;5(8):842–9.

31. Drilon AE, Sima CS, Somwar R, et al. Phase II study of cabozantinib for patients with advanced RET-rearranged lung cancers. ASCO Meet Abstr 2015;33(Suppl 15):8007.

32. Cappuzzo F, Bemis L, Varella-Garcia M. HER2 mutation and response to trastuzumab therapy in non-small-cell lung cancer. N Engl J Med 2006;354(24):2619–21.

33. Mazieres J, Peters S, Lepage B, et al. Lung cancer that harbors an HER2 mutation: epidemiologic characteristics and therapeutic perspectives. J Clin Oncol 2013;31(16):1997–2003.
34. Mellman I, Coukos G, Dranoff G. Cancer immunotherapy comes of age. Nature 2011;480(7378):480–9.
35. Rizvi NA, Mazieres J, Planchard D, et al. Activity and safety of nivolumab, an anti-PD-1 immune checkpoint inhibitor, for patients with advanced, refractory squamous non-small-cell lung cancer (CheckMate 063): a phase 2, single-arm trial. Lancet Oncol 2015;16(3):257–65.
36. Brahmer J, Reckamp KL, Baas P, et al. Nivolumab versus docetaxel in advanced squamous-cell non-small-cell lung cancer. N Engl J Med 2015;373(2):123–35.
37. Garon EB, Rizvi NA, Hui R, et al. Pembrolizumab for the treatment of non-small-cell lung cancer. N Engl J Med 2015;372(21):2018–28.
38. Schmidt LH, Kummel A, Gorlich D, et al. PD-1 and PD-L1 expression in NSCLC indicate a favorable prognosis in defined subgroups. PLoS One 2015;10(8): e0136023.
39. Liu SV, Powderly JD, Camidge DR, et al. Safety and efficacy of MPDL3280A (anti-PDL1) in combination with platinum-based doublet chemotherapy in patients with advanced non-small cell lung cancer (NSCLC). ASCO Meet Abstr 2015;33(Suppl 15):8030.
40. Lynch TJ, Bondarenko I, Luft A, et al. Ipilimumab in combination with paclitaxel and carboplatin as first-line treatment in stage IIIB/IV non-small-cell lung cancer: results from a randomized, double-blind, multicenter phase II study. J Clin Oncol 2012;30(17):2046–54.
41. Antonia SJ, Gettinger SN, Chow LQM, et al. Nivolumab (anti-PD-1; BMS-936558, ONO-4538) and ipilimumab in first-line NSCLC: interim phase I results. ASCO Meet Abstr 2014;32(Suppl 15):8023.

Local Therapy Indications in the Management of Patients with Oligometastatic Non–Small Cell Lung Cancer

Douglas A. Miller, MD*, Mark J. Krasna, MD

KEYWORDS

- Oligometastatic lung cancer • Intracranial radiosurgery
- Stereotactic ablative radiotherapy (SABR)

KEY POINTS

- Stereotactic ablative radiotherapy (SABR) carries the potential for durable local control of either solitary extrathoracic metastasis or persistent primary disease.
- Intracranial radiosurgery for small volume intracranial metastatic disease is the preferred first-line treatment at diagnosis for non–small cell lung cancer, with or without operative intervention.
- In absence of published randomized trials, the use of SABR in current clinical practice is most appropriately determined in the context of a multidisciplinary thoracic oncology team.

INTRODUCTION

From the very onset of an oncologist's clinical and specialty training, the concept of routine adherence to evidence-based medicine and clinical practice guidelines molds the physician to prescribe and administer therapy based on primary cancer site and stage. The oncologist follows established national and institutional pathways while simultaneously synthesizing the balance of documented disease presentation, patient age, performance status, and medical comorbidities to create a plan of care. Treatment is dynamically modified to disease response or progression, provided the patient remains an appropriate candidate for additional management. Successful eradication of disease earns professional and personal satisfaction, whereas progression of disease inherently necessitates the reevaluation of the therapeutic approach.

The rapid evolution of nontraditional treatments in the field of oncology medicine has afforded new opportunities for consideration of the inclusion of therapeutic

The authors have nothing to disclose.
Jersey Shore University Medical Center, Neptune, NJ 07753, USA
* Corresponding author.
E-mail address: DMiller@meridianhealth.com

approaches for isolated cancer lesions that extend beyond accepted guidelines and pathways. Minimally invasive surgical approaches, whether robot assisted or laparoscopic, often reduce the expected risks and complications previously considered barriers to their inclusion as part of cancer treatment. The evolution in clinical experience regarding the technical capabilities, applications, and toxicities for ablative radiotherapy to address specific sites of active disease remains an active area of clinical research and investigation. Radiofrequency or cryotherapy ablations offer additional opportunities for focused tissue destruction to address isolated foci of malignancy.

The oligometastatic disease state was first defined in 1995 and refers to a stage of disease, where cancer has spread beyond the site of origin, but is not yet widely metastatic.[1] In such a state of limited metastatic disease burden, it is hypothesized that eradication of all sites of metastatic disease could result in long-term survival, or even cure, in a subgroup of patients.[2] Ablation of metastatic deposits can be achieved surgically, or through stereotactic ablative radiotherapy (SABR), a new radiotherapy technology that delivers very large, hypofractionated doses of radiotherapy with high precision to small tumor targets, with high rates of local control.

Clinical evidence to support the presence of an oligometastatic state is emerging in both the surgical and SABR literature, for several tumor types. In a study of more than 5200 patients with lung metastases who underwent surgical resection, a 5-year survival of 36% was reported in patients who achieved a complete resection, which is much greater than would be expected for many patients with disseminated stage IV disease.[3] Similarly, in patients treated with SABR for 1 to 3 lung metastases from a variety of primary tumors types, local control with SABR was 96% at 2 years, and the 2-year survival was 39%.[4] The potential for long-term survival has been demonstrated in patients treated for oligometastases using surgery or SABR for metastatic lesions located in the liver, brain, bone, and adrenal glands. However, the risk of new metastatic disease, in either a new site or increase in clinical volume, remains high after ablative treatment, with reported rates up to 60% to 80%. Although SABR may be used as a further salvage treatment, often patient performance status and socioeconomic factors create functional limitations in the routine application for cancer treatment.

Despite the achievement of long-term survivors beyond statistical mean survivals with ablative treatment for oligometastatic disease, the level of evidence to support such treatments in routine clinical practice is weak in many cases, often based on single-arm studies without appropriate controls. The inclusion criteria for peer-reviewed publications show highly selected patients with good performance status and documented slow pace of tumor progression. Critics of ablative therapies have suggested that the long-term survival achieved by treatment of oligometastases is more a function of patient selection with slow tumor growth rather than the result of treatment intervention.[5]

Randomized trials are, therefore, necessary to establish the usefulness of ablative treatment of oligometastatic disease, but such randomized trials are rare. One such completed randomized trial, Radiation Therapy and Oncology Group Trial 9508, compared whole brain radiotherapy (WBRT) with WBRT plus stereotactic treatment for patients with 1 to 3 brain metastases, and found an overall survival advantage only in patients with a single metastasis and those patients in the most favorable baseline recursive partitioning analysis prognostic group. Patients with inferior baseline prognostic factors did not achieve a survival benefit from stereotactic boost treatment.[6]

It is unclear whether all patients with oligometastatic disease can benefit significantly from SABR, in terms of improved local control, improved survival, or improved quality of life. Although SABR generally results in successful ablation of each metastatic target, patients remain at high risk of further metastatic progression. Results from SABR for treatment of oligometastases in published studies appears promising, but these favorable results may be owing to patient selection, rather than treatment intervention, and are based on comparisons with historical controls. The benefit of comprehensive treatment of oligometastases can only be demonstrated conclusively in the context of a randomized trial.

Several ongoing studies are attempting to address these concerns, including the multicenter, Stereotactic Ablative Radiotherapy for Comprehensive Treatment of Oligometastatic Tumors (SABR-COMET) international study, which aims to accrue 99 patients and provide preliminary evidence to assess the impact of a comprehensive oligometastatic SABR treatment program on overall survival and quality of life. After stratification by the number of metastases (1–3 vs 4–5), patients will be randomized between arm 1 (current standard of care treatment) and arm 2 (standard of care treatment plus SABR to all sites of known disease; **Fig. 1**). For patients receiving

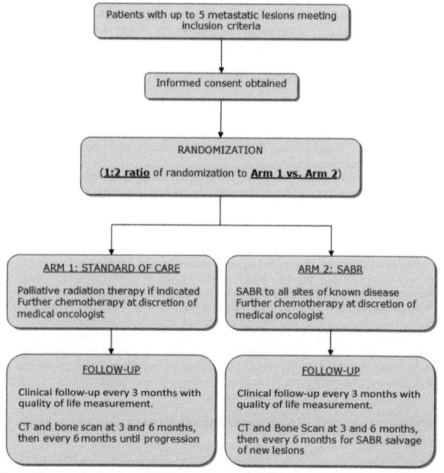

Fig. 1. Stereotactic Ablative Radiotherapy for Comprehensive Treatment of Oligometastatic Tumors (SABR-COMET) international randomized phase II study schema for patients with oligometastatic disease. CT, computed tomography.

SABR, radiotherapy dose and fractionation including motion management assessment is defined rigidly and based on location of metastasis and adjacent critical structure tolerances. The primary endpoint is overall survival, and secondary endpoints include quality of life, toxicity, progression-free survival, lesion control rate, and number of cycles of further chemotherapy/systemic therapy.[7]

This article touches on the clinical considerations and applications for the use of SABR with specific consideration for patients with oligometastatic non–small cell lung cancer (NSCLC).

STEREOTACTIC ABLATIVE RADIOTHERAPY TREATMENT PRINCIPLES

All patients receiving SABR should undergo treatment planning computed tomography (CT) simulation. Four-dimensional CT assessing the internal target volume should be strongly considered for thoracic or abdominal tumors. Axial CT images will be obtained throughout the region of interest. For all lesions, the gross tumor volume (GTV) will be defined as the visible tumor on pretreatment CT scan and/or MRI with or without PET. No additional margin is generally added to account for microscopic spread of disease, consistent with most radiosurgery current protocols (ie, clinical target volume = gross tumor volume). For vertebral lesions, the entire vertebral body may be considered the clinical target volume, as per institutional practice. A planning target volume (PTV) margin of 2 to 5 mm is added depending on the site of disease, methods of immobilization, and institutional setup accuracy. General considerations may include 2- to 3-mm margins may be used for spinal stereotactic treatments, 1 to 2 mm for brain tumors based on size of the intracranial lesion, and up to 5 mm for other sites. Organs at risk visible in the planning CT scan will be contoured. Constraints for 1-, 3-, and 5-fraction regimens are taken from Timmerman,[8] whereas equivalent doses were calculated for other fractionation schemes.

It is often recommended that dose constraints not be exceeded with specific attention to maximum point doses and absolute volume. If a dose constraint cannot be achieved owing to overlap of the target with an organ at risk, the fractionation can be increased or the target coverage compromised to meet the constraint. It is strongly recommended that in cases where the target coverage is compromised to meet the constraint, the mean dose delivered to the gross tumor volume should be at least 80% of the prescribed dose. Cases where a dose reduction or target coverage compromise often take into consideration prior radiation therapy, surgical treatment, or systemic therapy options. For most tumor sites, doses are prescribed to approximately the 100% isodose level and 95% of the PTV should receive 95% of the prescription dose. Doses should be corrected for tissue inhomogeneity.

For treatment delivery, cone-beam CT or other stereoscopic imaging capability should be used to verify patient positioning immediately before treatment (**Fig. 2**). Ideally, direct target localization should be performed for stereotactic treatments of soft tissues with consideration of intrafraction target volume identification using fiducial markers or specialized tracking software.

STEREOTACTIC ABLATIVE RADIOTHERAPY FOR THE MANAGEMENT OF VISCERAL METASTASES

Although we await the results of randomized trials to determine the benefits of ablative treatment for oligometastatic NSCLC, treatment decisions for such patients need to be made in the interim, and such decisions can be informed by other levels of evidence. Oligometastatic NSCLC remains a common topic of investigation for the

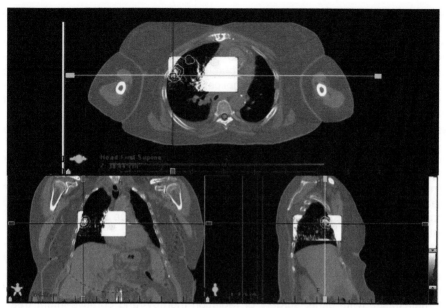

Fig. 2. Cone-beam computed tomography (CT) localization for lung metastasis treated with SABR. Patient is rigidly immobilized, and pretreatment imaging is obtained to localize the dense lesion at cross-hairs within the right lung. The newly acquired CT images (*small highlighted rectangle*) are matched to full body planning CT simulation in 3 planes: axial (*top*), coronal (*bottom, left*) and sagittal (*bottom, right*) before treatment.

improved control of visceral metastases, in both the radiation oncology and the surgery literature. With no clear standardized approach, a comprehensive review of all reports and applications of SABR in clinical practice exceeds the scope of this article. In summary, SABR routinely provides local control rates between 80% to 90% of disease defined by a treated field regardless of anatomic location. The variability of SABR dosing regimens, use of concurrent systemic agents (eg cytotoxic or biological therapy), and prior interventions before SABR prevent the publication of a specified treatment regimen or inclusion point for SABR in patient care pathway. Best practice guidelines advocate that in patients with oligometastatic NSCLC, a multi-disciplinary approach to identify sequencing of therapy and benefits of SABR be thoroughly discussed before use.

A single-arm phase II trial reported by Iyengar and colleagues[9] enrolled patients with stage IV NSCLC and 6 or more sites of extracranial disease, with a maximum of 3 pulmonary or 3 liver lesions. Early chemotherapy had failed in all the patients, and they had received SABR to all sites of disease with concurrent erlotinib (150 mg/d starting 1 week before SABR and continued until disease progression). Epidermal growth factor receptor testing was not mandatory at enrollment. Acceptable SABR doses allowed for physician discretion and included treatment regimens of 19 to 24 Gy in 1 fraction, 27 to 33 Gy in 3 fractions, or 35 to 40 Gy in 5 fractions, all considered radiobiologically equivalent. Patients who developed disease progression after SABR were allowed to remain in the trial and continue erlotinib if the new lesions were outside the previously radiated field and amenable to additional SABR. The primary endpoint was 6-month progression-free survival. A total of 24 patients were accrued and 52 lesions treated, most commonly in the lung (18 lesions) or mediastinum/hilum (13 lesions). Of the 24 patients, 13 underwent epidermal growth factor receptor mutation testing, all with negative results. The mean follow-up period was 16.8 months. Regarding SABR-related toxicity, 1 grade 5 toxicity developed that was possibly attributable to radiation (acute respiratory distress syndrome or pneumonia after SABR to 3 thoracic targets), 1 grade 4 event in the same patient, and 2 patients with grade 3 complications (radiation pneumonitis and vertebral compression fracture). The trial met its primary endpoint, with a 69% rate of 6-month progression-free survival. The median overall survival was 20.4 months. Most treatment failures were at distant sites, with only 3 local failures of 47 evaluable lesions treated with SABR (crude rate 6%). In contrast, 10 patients experienced failure with new metastases outside the treated fields. The main conclusions from their trial are that the progression-free survival and overall survival outcomes are promising with this approach. The successful ablation of all metastatic deposits changes the pattern of progression, with a shift from progression at existing sites of disease to progression at new sites of disease, some of which might be amenable to further SABR.

An individual patient data metaanalysis of outcomes and prognostic factors after treatment of oligometastatic NSCLC assessed individual patient data from 757 patients with oligometastatic NSCLC from 20 centers.[10] All patients had 1 to 5 synchronous or metachronous oligometastases and were treated with ablation of all metastases (with either surgery or radiation therapy) and curative-intent treatment of the primary tumor. The data were divided into separate training and validation datasets, and recursive partitioning analysis was used to create the risk groups.

Patients included in the metaanalysis were highly selected with low-burden disease: 88% had only 1 metastasis, nearly two-thirds harbored intrathoracic stage I or II disease, and 98% had a good performance status. Overall, with a median follow-up period of 53 months, the 1- and 5-year overall survival rates were 70% and 29%, respectively. In the training set, the factors predictive of improved overall survival on Cox multivariable analysis were metachronous presentation (vs synchronous), lower N stage, and adenocarcinoma histologic type. On recursive partitioning analysis, the patients were divided into 3 groups: low risk (patients with metachronous presentation, 5-year overall survival 48%), intermediate risk (patients with synchronous presentation and N0 disease, 5-year overall survival 36%), and high risk (patients with synchronous presentation and higher N stage disease, 5-year overall survival 14%). The results from both the Cox analysis and the recursive partitioning analysis remained significant in the validation set. The results suggest that the most important factors influencing survival seem to relate to indolent tumor biology, metachronous presentation, and the absence of nodal metastases rather than treatment factors. It is evident that some highly selected patients, particularly those in the low-risk group, can achieve excellent long-term outcomes. Such a stratification schema could be useful for informing the design of future trials.

These analyses are representative of the increasing body of evidence suggesting that a substantial number of patients with oligometastatic NSCLC can achieve a long disease-free interval after ablative treatments, supporting the rationale for ongoing clinical trials. Although the outcomes in these single-arm studies seem to be promising, some caution is warranted. Observational data alone showing "better-than-expected" outcomes can lead to erroneous conclusions, such as was demonstrated by the premature adoption of high-dose chemotherapy followed by hematopoietic stem cell transplant for metastatic breast cancer in the 1980s.[11]

Many questions remain, including the influence of tumor biology, which biomarkers will be useful, and the effect of novel systemic therapies. Variations in metastatic potential based on tumor biology could have profound implications on the chances of further distant relapse. Clinically useful biomarkers to distinguish between potential for oligometastatic versus polymetastatic disease have yet to be defined. The importance of effective systemic therapy to address occult micrometastases in patients with oligometastatic disease has long been recognized. Emerging therapies (eg, targeted agents or immunotherapy) might better address occult micrometastases, decreasing the risk of distant failure. In such a scenario, with better control of micrometastases, achieving local control of known oligometastatic deposits with radiation therapy or surgery would be expected to have a larger effect on overall survival.

STEREOTACTIC RADIOSURGERY FOR MANAGEMENT OF BRAIN METASTASES

Metastasis of a primary tumor to the brain is a common problem, affecting on the order of 200,000 cancer patients in the United States each year. Traditional management of brain metastases includes a clinical decision between traditional WBRT or stereotactic radiosurgery (SRS), either alone or in combination with WBRT. With all forms of radiation therapy, the challenge is to deliver an adequate dose to kill all tumor cells while minimizing the dose to surrounding normal tissue. In SRS, the balance of tumor destruction and normal tissue preservation is achieved by precisely and accurately delivering a very high dose of radiation in 1 or a few fractions to a limited, well-defined volume (**Fig. 3**).

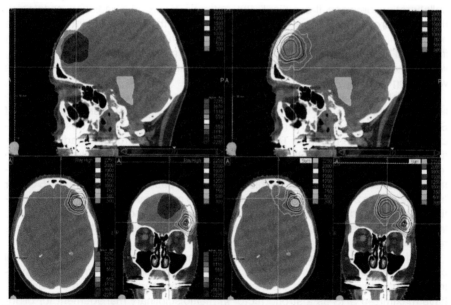

Fig. 3. Stereotactic radiosurgery uses a high degree of accuracy and treatment planning to minimize toxicity while providing durable local control. The patient in **Fig. 2** developed a new inferior left frontal 1.4 cm brain lesion (*yellow*) in the same lobe as a previously treated solitary anterior frontal brain metastasis (*blue, top, left*) 9 months earlier. Successful control of the second lesion was obtained without dosimetry overlap (*bottom, far right*), and the patient continues to be free of intracranial disease 18 months out from initial diagnosis and presentation.

With appropriate quality assurance, the precision and accuracy of intracranial SRS does not compromise local control. It has been hypothesized that there is a very low number of tumor cells extending beyond the visible periphery of the lesion, the radiation dose in the periphery is adequate to kill microscopic peritumoral disease, or both. A recent randomized trial by Kirkpatrick and colleagues[12] assessed the adequacy of small margin PTV expansion and impact on radiosurgery efficacy and toxicity. Forty-nine patients with 80 brain metastases were treated with SRS using a PTV expansion of 1 or 3 mm. The median overall survival was 10.6 months, and local control of the treated tumor regardless of initial treatment size was 93.3%. Further, 3 months after SRS, no change in neurocognition or quality of life was observed. The conclusion that a 1-mm margin expansion seems to offer high rates of local control and minimal morbidity in the setting of a dedicated radiosurgery system, high-resolution imaging, and a robust quality assurance program has been translated to many current clinical practices.

Rates of local recurrence after SRS are low based on reports of prospective trials (**Table 1**). The issue of SRS alone versus WBRT versus SRS and WBRT in combination is controversial. Clearly, WBRT reduces the rate of distant brain metastases after a "local" therapy such as SRS or surgical resection, but the net benefits in terms of overall survival, preservation of neurocognition, and quality of life have not been established. Although several studies support the observation that patients treated with radiosurgery alone can achieve high rates of local control, the rate of distant brain metastases is high, and it is unknown which patients would benefit from the addition of WBRT to SRS to reduce distant brain failures. There will always be a continuous need for close follow-up and for ongoing, effective collaboration between the patient, the patient's family, the radiation oncologist, the neurosurgeon, and other caregivers. Further, in the posttreatment surveillance of patients, the clinical decision to consider additional SRS based on follow-up imaging is important. Often salvage SRS for 1 or 2 new lesions may be appropriate, whereas a higher number of lesions suggest untreated micrometastatic disease warranting WBRT.

The safety of SRS has been well-established in prospective clinical trials and published reports. Unlike the heterogeneity in applications and regimens for the use of SABR for visceral lesions, the management and maximum tolerated doses for intracranial SRS has been defined. The principles of SRS derived from the Radiation Therapy Oncology Group (RTOG) 90-05 protocol remain in widespread clinical adoption for intracranial dose and fractionation.[13] The maximum tolerated doses of single fraction radiosurgery were defined for this population of patients as 24, 18, and 15 Gy for tumors less than 20 mm, 21 to 30 mm, and 31 to 40 mm in maximum diameter, respectively. Unacceptable central nervous system toxicity was more likely in patients with larger tumors, whereas local tumor control was more dependent on the type of recurrent tumor.

SRS for intracranial disease remains a safe and effective option for durable local control of oligometastatic disease to the brain. Evolution of pretreatment imaging, along with a reduction in uncertainties associated with treatment delivery have maximized SRS as a strong factor in multidisciplinary management for oligometastatic patients. The classic recursive partitioning analysis stratification suggesting a mean survival of 7 months for the only the "healthiest" of patients with brain metastasis continues to shift in a positive direction. The potential for longer term durable control of intracranial disease ultimately affords the clinician the opportunity to evaluate other therapies and modalities to improve disease free and overall survival.

Table 1
Median overall survival, local failure, and distant brain metastasis rates of 4 randomized trials using SRS as primary treatment for intracranial disease

Study	No. of Patients	No. of Lesions	GTV to PTV Expansion	Rate of Local Recurrence 1 y After SRS, %	Rate of Distant Brain Metastases 1 y After SRS, %	Median Overall Survival After SRS, mo (/TH)
JRSOG 99–1	67	101–165[a]	None	28	76	8.0
M D Anderson	30	47	None	33	73	15.6
EORTC 22952–26001	90	128	1–2 mm	29	42	10.7
Duke (this study)	49	80	1 or 3 mm	7	46	10.6

Abbreviations: EORTC, European Organisation for Research and Treatment of Cancer; GTV, gross tumor volume; JROSG, Japanese Radiation Oncology Study Group; PTV, planning target volume; SRS, stereotactic radiosurgery.

[a] Based on reported 33 patients with 1 brain lesion and 34 patients with 2 to 4 brain lesions.

From Kirkpatrick JP, Wang Z, Sampson JH, et al. Defining the optimal planning target volume in image-guided stereotactic radiosurgery of brain metastases: results of a randomized trial. Int J Radiat Oncol Biol Phys 2015;91(1):100–8; with permission.

SUMMARY

In current clinical practice, the diagnosis of oligometastatic disease remains a tremendous enigma in oncology care. The clinician must struggle to balance the science of the disease—the purest form of the word incurable—with the compassion of direct human care and personalized medicine to afford a patient the opportunity of long-term "cure." Fortunately, the continued development of novel surgical techniques, targeted chemo/bio therapeutics and technological advancements with SABR/SRS offer a potential avenue to achieve what in today's understanding would be considered unachievable.

ACKNOWLEDGMENTS

This article is dedicated to our patients.

REFERENCES

1. Hellman S, Weichselbaum R. Oligometastases. J Clin Oncol 1995;13(1):8–10.
2. Macdermed DM, Weichselbaum RR, Salama JK. A rationale for the targeted treatment of oligometastases with radiotherapy. J Surg Oncol 2008;98(3):202–6.
3. Pastorino U, Buyse M, Friedel G, et al. Long-term results of lung metastasectomy: prognostic analyses based on 5206 cases. Metastases., The International Registry of Lung. J Thorac Cardiovasc Surg 1997;113(1):37–49.
4. Rusthoven KE, Kavanagh BD, Burri SH, et al. Multi-institutional phase I/II trial of stereotactic body radiation therapy for lung metastases. J Clin Oncol 2009;27(10):1579–84.
5. Primrose J, Treasure T, Fiorentino F. Lung metastasectomy in colorectal cancer: is this surgery effective in prolonging life? Respirology 2010;15(5):742–6.
6. Andrews DW, Scott CB, Sperduto PW, et al. Whole brain radiation therapy with or without stereotactic radiosurgery boost for patients with one to three brain metastases: phase III results of the RTOG 9508 randomised trial. Lancet 2004;363(9422):1665–72.
7. Palma DA, Haasbeek CJA, Rodrigues GB, et al. Stereotactic ablative radiotherapy for comprehensive treatment of oligometastatic tumors (SABR-COMET): Study protocol for a randomized phase II trial. BMC Cancer 2012;12:305.
8. Timmerman RD. An Overview of Hypofractionation and Introduction to This Issue of Seminars in Radiation Oncology. Semin Radiat Oncol 2008;18(4):215–22.
9. Iyengar P, Kavanagh BD, Wardak Z, et al. Phase II trial of stereotactic body radiation therapy combined with erlotinib for patients with limited but progressive metastatic non–small-cell lung cancer. J Clin Oncol 2014;32:3824–30.
10. Ashworth AB, Senan S, Palma DA, et al. An individual patient data metaanalysis of outcomes and prognostic factors after treatment of oligometastatic non-small-cell lung cancer. Clin Lung Cancer 2014;15:346–55.
11. Palma DA, Salama JK, Lo SS, et al. The oligometastatic state- separating truth from wishful thinking. Nat Rev Clin Oncol 2014;11:549–57.
12. Kirkpatrick JP, Wang Z, Sampson JH, et al. Defining the optimal planning target volume in image-guided stereotactic radiosurgery of brain metastases: results of a randomized trial. Int J Radiat Oncol Biol Phys 2015;91(1):100–8.
13. Shaw E, Scott C, Souhami L, et al. Single dose radiosurgical treatment of recurrent previously irradiated primary brain tumors and brain metastases: final report of RTOG protocol 90-05. Int J Radiat Oncol Biol Phys 2000;47(2):291–8.

Printed and bound by CPI Group (UK) Ltd, Croydon, CR0 4YY

13/10/2024

01773593-0001